Developmental Theory and Language Disorders

Trends in Language Acquisition Research

Official publication of the International Association for the Study of Child Language (IASCL).

IASCL website: http://atila-www.uia.ac.be/IASCL

Volume 4

Developmental Theory and Language Disorders
Edited by Paul Fletcher and Jon F. Miller

Developmental Theory and Language Disorders

Edited by

Paul Fletcher

University College Cork

Jon F. Miller

University of Wisconsin-Madison

John Benjamins Publishing Company

Amsterdam / Philadelphia

∞™ The paper used in this publication meets the minimum requirements of American National Standard for Information Sciences – Permanence of Paper for Printed Library Materials, ANSI Z39.48-1984.

Library of Congress Cataloging-in-Publication Data

Developmental Theory and Language Disorders / edited by Paul Fletcher and Jon F. Miller.
p. cm. (Trends in Language Acquisition Research, ISSN 1569–0644 ; v. 4)
Includes bibliographical references and index.
Contents: Developmental theory and language disorders / Jon Miller and Paul Fletcher -- Constraints on language development / Michael S.C. Thomas -- Constructions and language development / Paul Fletcher, Stephanie Stokes, and Anita Wong -- Language development in Down syndrome and fragile X syndrome / Leonard Abbeduto and Robin S. Chapman -- The role of language and communication impairments within autism / Morten Ann Gernsbacher, Heather M. Greye, and Ellis Weismer -- Language acquisition in children with a cochlear implant / Karen Schauwers, Steven Gilles, and Paul Govaerts -- Critical periods in the acquisition of lexical skills / Amy R. Lederberg and Patricia E. Spencer -- Developmental theory and language disorders / Michael Garman, Deborah James, and Vesna Stojanovik.
1. Language acquisition. 2. Language disorders. I. Fletcher, Paul (Paul J.). II. Miller, Jon F. III. Series.

P118.D476 2005
401'.93--dc22 2005040617
ISBN 90 272 3474 4 (Eur.) / 1 58811 631 X (US) (Hb; alk. paper)

John Benjamins Publishing Co. · P.O. Box 36224 · 1020 ME Amsterdam · The Netherlands
John Benjamins North America · P.O. Box 27519 · Philadelphia PA 19118-0519 · USA

Table of contents

List of contributors

Leonard Abbeduto
Waisman Center
University of Wisconsin-Madison
USA

Robin Chapman
Waisman Center
University of Wisconsin-Madison
USA

Susan Ellis Weismer
Department of Communicative Disorders and Waisman Center
University of Wisconsin-Madison
USA

Paul Fletcher
Department of Speech and Hearing Sciences
University College Cork
Ireland

Michael Garman
School of Linguistics and Applied Language Studies
University of Reading
UK

Morton Ann Gernsbacher
Department of Psychology and Waisman Center
University of Wisconsin-Madison
USA

Heather M. Geye
Department of Psychology and Waisman Center
University of Wisconsin-Madison
USA

Steven Gillis
CNTS – Department of Linguistics
University of Antwerp
Belgium

Paul Govaerts
The Eargroup, Antwerp-Deurne
Belgium

Deborah James
School of Education, Communication and Language Sciences
University of Newcastle-upon-Tyne
UK

Amy R. Lederberg
Department of Educational Psychology and Special Education
Georgia State University
USA

Jon Miller
Department of Communicative Disorders and Waisman Center
University of Wisconsin-Madison
USA

Karen Schauwers
CNTS – Department of Linguistics
University of Antwerp and
The Eargroup, Antwerp-Deurne
Belgium

Patricia E. Spencer
Department of Social Work
Gallaudet University
USA

Vesna Stojanovik
School of Linguistics and
Applied Language Studies
University of Reading
UK

Stephanie Stokes
School of Linguistics and
Applied Language Studies
University of Reading
UK

Michael S. C. Thomas
School of Psychology
Birkbeck College
University of London
UK

Anita M.-Y. Wong
Division of Speech and Hearing Sciences
University of Hong Kong
Hong Kong
China

Preface

The present volume is the fourth in the series 'Trends in Language Acquisition Research' (TiLAR). As an official publication of the *International Association for the Study of Child Language* (IASCL), the TiLAR Series publishes two volumes per three year period in between IASCL congresses. All volumes in the IASCL-TiLAR Series are invited edited volumes by IASCL members that are strongly thematic in nature and that present cutting edge work which is likely to stimulate further research to the fullest extent.

Besides quality, diversity is also an important consideration in all the volumes and in the series as a whole: diversity of theoretical and methodological approaches, diversity in the languages studied, diversity in the geographical and academic backgrounds of the contributors. After all, like the IASCL itself, the IASCL-TiLAR Series is there for child language researchers from all over the world.

After the previous volumes, on bilingual acquisition, sign language acquisition, and language development beyond the early childhood years, respectively, we now are very pleased to present the current volume on child language disorders and how these inform developmental theory or are informed by it. We are very grateful to the volume editors, Paul Fletcher and Jon Miller, for their willingness to contribute their long-standing expertise in this area. They have brought together an impressive collection of state-of-the-art work by leading scholars from a variety of backgrounds. We hope this volume can indeed help to bridge the gap that often exists between researchers in the more applied communication disorders field and those working in more theoretically oriented disciplines.

We would like to thank Seline Benjamins and Kees Vaes of John Benjamins Publishing Company for their trust and their concerted efforts in helping to make important deadlines. We also thank the TiLAR Advisory Board for this volume, viz. IASCL past presidents Jean Berko Gleason, Ruth Berman, Philip Dale, and Brian MacWhinney, for their much appreciated advice.

'Trends in Language Acquisition Research' is made for and by IASCL members, and an integral benefit of IASCL membership. We hope that the series is a meaningful and important source of information and inspiration to the community of child language researchers all over the world.

Antwerp, October 2004
The General Editors

Developmental theory and language disorders

Background issues

Jon Miller and Paul Fletcher

1. Introduction

In the summer of 2002 a unique conference took place in Madison, Wisconsin (U.S.A.), under the auspices of the University of Wisconsin and the International Association for the Study of Child Language. In a week-long joint meeting, the International Association for the Study of Child Language, and the Symposium for Research in Child Language Disorders, joined forces. These two groups had previously met separately. The IASCL grew out of a meeting held on language acquisition in Florence, Italy, in 1972, and has been coming together at different venues around the world every three years since then. The SRCLD since its inception in 1980 has met annually in Madison. Common membership between the groups, and common interests in typical and atypical language acquisition, have always seen cross-fertilization. The 2002 joint meeting was designed to build on these informal links and to take advantage of the occasion to explore in detail the interaction between developmental theory and developmental language disorders. The intent of this volume is to archive a number of papers presented at the IASCL/SRCLD meeting that are relevant to this relationship in identified populations. At the 2002 meeting, state-of-the-art research findings were presented from children with hearing impairment, children with developmental disabilities, e.g., autism, and mental retardation, and children with specific language impairment (SLI). The chapters in this volume summarize the research on specific populations and address the general question of how data from these populations inform theories of language acquisition. A final chapter identifies themes that emerge across the chapters.

Language disorder is here considered from a broad perspective, including children with language disorder with no identifiable cause (SLI) as well as children with a variety of developmental disabilities, including mental retardation, autism and deafness. This scope provides an exploration of the many ways in which language disorder manifests itself, as well as the opportunity to consider how various developmental outcomes can be explained by contemporary developmental theory, variations on innateness or environmental input.

A range of questions arise. Can the language performance of children with SLI be explained by the absence of specific language modules, as for instance, the ability to learn rules, or by a generally less efficient language processing system? Why do children with SLI fail to grow out of their language problems? And what is the significance of their difficulty for the acquisition of literacy skills? Are oral language and reading difficulty related? Do children with developmental disabilities have unique profiles of development? Do children with unique brain syndromes have unique profiles of development? Do children with different etiologies have different profiles of strengths and weaknesses? How do language profiles change through the developmental period? Is there evidence for critical periods of development? Does language continue to develop beyond the typical developmental period? Is language disorder realized similarly for children learning a variety of languages? These and other questions are addressed in the chapters that follow. While each chapter was written independently, and the chapters focus on different populations, consistent themes emerge.

As the chapters in this volume unfold, the polarity of the theoretical positions, nature versus nurture, becomes refocused from various perspectives. Neurologically, the issue can be formulated in terms of the brain having a specific language learning organ as opposed to a language learning mechanism made up of spare parts (Bates 2004). Linguistically, the search is for the specific area or areas of the grammar in which difficulties are manifest, and then for what can be inferred from any identified faultlines about the source of the problem(s). Developmentally, the concern is to determine whether patterns of performance observed early in development are or are not sustained through life.

A language disorder is defined relative to a reference, either chronological age (CA) or mental age (MA). Mental age is generally measured with non-verbal tests or sub-tests taken from intelligence batteries. Non-verbal mental age has been shown to be highly correlated with developing language milestones in children with mental retardation with a variety of syndromes (Abbeduto 2003). The issue of the standard for judging typical or non-typical performance is particularly relevant for considering severity. Should severity be a matter of degree, e.g., standard deviations below CA or MA, the number of language areas affected (phonology, syntax, semantics, pragmatics), or the modes affected (comprehension and production, or production only)? While answers to all of these questions may not be found in this volume, certainly they provide the framework through which to assess the state of the science on the nature of language disorder and its relation and contribution to developmental theory.

In the remainder of this introductory chapter we will look more closely at the background to studies on SLI, and studies on developmental disabilities with identified etiologies. There is a striking contrast to be noted between work on SLI, which seeks causal constructs that are frequently drawn from developmental theory or theories, and research on children with identified etiologies, which seems to have description as its main focus. Identified etiologies define the cause of problems, and research centers on the consequence for speech, language and communication skills. Research on SLI must define the problem, the nature of the language performance that classifies the child as impaired, and then examine the cognitive abilities, environmental mechanisms and contextual sensitivities of these children. A closer look at each research approach will illuminate their similarities and differences.

2. Specific language impairment

The research on children with SLI identifies a variety of causal constructs for their language impairment. From a non-nativist perspective these may include information processing deficits, specific cognitive skill deficits, poor working memory and phonological awareness deficits. Alternatively, on the nativist view, impairments may be focused on grammar itself. This may involve difficulty in establishing structural relationships in sentences, a plateau of development where marking tense is optional, or a general difficulty in learning implicit rules. The range of these explanations may be due to a number of issues, from differences in the underlying theory to variation in subjects participating in each study.

Children with SLI participating in research studies are generally identified by the researchers. In most cases participants are receiving services, but this tends not to be a defining characteristic. The variability in participants may be traced to four issues. The first issue involves inclusion criteria for enrolling children with SLI and control groups. The second related issue concerns the tests of language performance themselves and their ability to identify children with SLI, distinguishing them from typical children. The third issue concerns the reference point for categorizing children as disordered, the gold standard. The final issue concerns the homogeneity of the target population: are children with SLI a single group of children defined by the same comprehension and production criteria, or are there subgroups of children with specific profiles of language difficulties, e.g., word finding problems or utterance formulation problems?

2.1 Inclusion criteria

A review of research on children with SLI published over the past two years explored subject inclusion criteria for children with SLI (Heilmann 2004). These criteria can be taken as definitions for SLI, because the results are generalized to the SLI population.

Thirty-six studies were published in 2003–2004 on SLI in English. Sample sizes range from 2 to 158, with an average of about 26 participants. Ages ranged from 3.2–15.4 years but studies usually focused on a restricted range, e.g., 4–5, 4–6, 8–12. Studies generally considered SLI as a single group, with no subgroups mentioned in 26 studies. Socio-economic status was provided in only 9 studies, with 27 studies providing no SES data. General trends in language test performance revealed 22 studies with specific criteria from standardized language assessments and/or language sample analysis, but a surprising 14 studies gave no specific criteria. Test criteria ranged from –1 SD in nine studies, to –1.25 SDs in two studies, to –1.5 SDs in nine studies. One study used 'less than the tenth percentile' as its inclusion criterion. One study used an age discrepancy of 11 months to identify subjects and the final study employed a test discrepancy of 25 points. Twelve studies used either comprehensive tests or a combination of tests with criteria ranging from –1 SD to –1.5 SDs, five studies used a combination of receptive and expressive scores, with four of these five studies using –1 SD as criterion for inclusion. Thirty one out of 36 studies mention cognitive criteria. These range from a blanket statement of 'within normal limits', to a score above the 10th percentile, to IQ scores in the range of 70 to 85, to scores above 85 (that is above –1 SD).

The spread of criteria characterizing SLI which is apparent in these recent research studies suggests that at the very least the severity of language impairment is quite variable. It could be argued that many of these studies were studying children at the low end of the normal distribution. The only long term investigation of a relatively large group of children identified as SLI comes from

Tomblin and colleagues' Iowa Language Disorders research project where the participants were identified at kindergarten from a randomized sample of several thousand typical children using very explicit criteria (Tomblin, Records, Buckwalter, Zhang, Smith, & O'Brien 1997). Studies of children proposed to be SLI should not be compared unless the subject samples can be shown to come from the same population of children.

2.2 Selectivity and sensitivity of language tests

There are several things to mention here, including the type of test, and knowledge versus processes related to language learning. Several studies document the sensitivity of process tests like non-word repetition tests (Dollaghan & Campbell 1998). Plante and Vance (1994) document the relatively poor sensitivity and selectivity data on most standardized tests in English. Data on criterion reference measures like MLU show sensitivity/selectivity rates as high as many standardized tests (Dunn, Flax, Slivinski, & Aram 1996). Miller, Lall, Hollar, Jones, Lodholtz, Pech, Rolland, Tarnow, Vernon, Wood and Dagget (2001) document selectivity/sensitivity rates of 79/86% for a group of measures derived from language samples: MLU, number of different words, speaking rate and fluency. A number of investigators are working on new tests that show improved selectivity/sensitivity outcomes (Rice & Wexler 2001; Gillam & Pearson 2004; Peña, Gutierrez-Clellen, Iglesias, Goldstein, Bedore in preparation; Seymour, Roeper, & de Villiers 2003). Documenting the sensitivity and selectivity of a test requires agreement on who has a language disorder. This requires agreement on the definition and the standards for the measurement of language knowledge and/or language processes. Issues of severity as well as onset and developmental change must be considered, as well as the longitudinal outcome of the disorder.

2.3 The gold standard

It is generally agreed that children with SLI have delayed onset and protracted language development, but other exclusionary criteria, including IQ and neurological impairment require further study (Tager-Flusberg & Cooper 1999). Typically, test scores are used with standard score criteria cited, i.e., a knowledge based assessment is used, but there is an increasing body of work suggesting that process assessments should be included in defining the disorder as well, such as non-word repetition tasks (Dollaghan & Campbell 1998). The comparison groups for either of these measurements are typical children meeting standardization criteria for tests and criterion reference data from experimental work. Alternatively, children could be compared to other family members in terms of volubility, rate of speaking and other measures of linguistic flexibility given the work of Hart and Risley (1992, 1995). This ground breaking work found that children closely resembled their parents in their language facility and that the amount of talking directed to children predicted the rate of language development. More talk resulted in children who not only talked more but who also used more complex language. Huttenlocher and colleagues found similar outcomes in experimental studies of typical children (Huttenlocher, Haight, & Bryk 1991; Huttenlocher, Vasilyeva, Cymerman, & Levine 2002).

It is interesting to note that most researchers find it very difficult to find children with SLI who meet the accepted definition of the disorder. As little as 10% of the case load of American school speech and language pathologists may qualify, even though in an American state like Wisconsin, the criteria for receiving services is –1.75 standard deviations on standardized measures. Differences in subject inclusion criteria for research and criteria for qualifying for services in the schools are generally not discussed, or are evaluated relative to generalizing research findings.

2.4 SLI sub-types

Children with SLI are viewed as having expressive deficits only, or as having both receptive and expressive deficits. The additional components of phonological deficits and reduced speech intelligibility are also recognized. Studies published over the last few years tend to delineate these groups of children. Recognition of a semantic-pragmatic disorder has prompted some investigators to specifically exclude these children (Bishop 2004). Another group of children who are considered to be language impaired, but not usually mentioned in participant inclusion criteria, are children with word finding problems. One wonders how many of these children meet the inclusion criteria of published research studies or whether they exhibit different language profiles. Given the small sample size of most studies, the question is how similar these children are on measures of verbal fluency, i.e., repetitions and revisions that characterize word finding problems, or talkativeness in general, e.g., children who produce less talk per unit time, a measure linked to general language proficiency (Iglesias 2004).

In summary, the research on SLI over the past two years tends to view children with SLI as a single group, is focused on central tendencies, and explains away performance variability.

When we consider the cross-linguistic work, these issues take on new significance as different languages appear to produce different behavioral phenotypes. Clearly cross-linguistic work examining children who are learning a wide variety of languages and studies of SLI suggests that the specific language being learned has an influence on the manifestation of disordered performance (see Leonard 1998). This should perhaps not be surprising, but it does introduce another level of complexity to the puzzle of characterizing language disorder.

3. Language in children with developmental disabilities

Are there unique brain syndromes associated with specific developmental disabilities that cause particular difficulties with language learning and use? Research on the language and communication abilities of children with mental retardation has a long history. The modern era of theory driven work began at the University of Kansas in the 1950s based on B. F. Skinner's research using operant conditioning paradigms (Skinner 1957). The Kansas research group was interested in using operant conditioning as a means of studying learning in general as well as speech and language behavior in moderate to profoundly mentally retarded children. In addition, the group was interested in developing methods to improve these children's speech, language and communication. Their research assumed that any child could learn any behavior if the behavior was broken down into its component parts in small enough units and presented in the appropriate sequence for mastery. Teaching speech became an effort of shaping articulation through experimenter stimulus presentation, child response and experimenter reinforcement. In theory, behaviors would repeat if appropriately reinforced. Learning could be entirely explained by environmental factors, while cognition and intellectual function were products of learning rather than the driving force. This work ultimately demonstrated that children who were moderately and even severely retarded could learn almost anything in the laboratory given enough trials. Learning was defined as producing the appropriate response to the experimental stimuli. The issue that plagued this work was the generalization of learning: Children could not make use of their new behaviors in new situations in the laboratory or their daily lives. It seems obvious now that the lack of generalization can be explained as the expected result of teaching behaviors without developmental reference, i.e., mental age reflecting general knowledge of the world, and in isolation, i.e., outside of their functional contexts.

In the 1970s, research on language development was documenting the uniqueness of language learning where children were constructing grammars seemingly on their own, and producing sentences that could not have been heard in their environment. As development progressed, these grammars were being re-organized to adult status (Bloom 1970; Brown 1973). This work prompted researchers to reconsider language behavior in developmental terms rather than in terms of stimulus- response paradigms. Documented sequences of language development allowed researchers to evaluate the language and communication of children classified as mentally retarded to determine if their spontaneous language was a unique form of English, or whether it followed the same sequence as typical children, but at a slower rate: Do significant differences in intellectual function result in language that is 'deviant', or merely delayed? The results of this work generally supported the delayed development perspective, while researchers continued to struggle with the issue of what constituted 'deviant' language. New approaches to intervention began to emerge (Miller & Yoder 1972, 1974), which invoked developmental sequences as the bases of selecting learning targets for syntactic teaching programs. The idea was to promote learning by selecting learning targets at, or slightly above, the child's current level of development. These programs emphasized developmental appropriateness as well as functional utility in the identification of intervention targets.

In the 1970s a series of volumes were published summarizing the research on language development in children with mental retardation from these diverse theoretical perspectives (Schiefelbusch 1972; Mclean, Yoder, & Schiefelbusch 1972; Schiefelbusch & Lloyd 1974). This work recognized that mental retardation is a behavioral classification, characterized by levels of retardation – mild, moderate, severe and profound – without reference to specific etiologies, genetic or brain syndromes. This view reflected the fact that at the time, only about 30% of individuals classified as mentally retarded had an identified etiology that allowed them to be considered as one group. Today, almost 80% of those classified as mentally retarded have an identified etiology. It is now understood that language evolves in the same sequence as in typically developing children, but that there are unique differences in the language outcomes for children with different etiologies. Even the most profoundly retarded person has some form of communication (McLean & Cripe 1997) and children who never experience a language in their environment can create a language system (Goldin-Meadow 2002). Clearly children bring a great deal to the language learning task, but what features are "hard wired" versus shaped by experience is a topic that continues to be explored by the chapters in this volume.

Research through the 1990s began to focus on specific etiologies in which language and communication skills did not follow the pattern of extended normal development. Theoretical debates were fueled by descriptions of children with severe hydrocephalus (Cromer 1994) and children with Williams Syndrome arguing that despite their severe mental retardation, these children's language was spared, and functioning at near normal levels (Pinker 1994; Smith & Tsimpli 1995; Piattelli-Palmarini 2001). This debate continues today, but focuses on specific linguistic features such as syntax, vocabulary, and discourse, rather than on global language performance. Furthermore, there are a number of studies whose results are at odds with the view that language is spared in Williams syndrome, and that find that language generally follows mental age development (Bates 2004; Reilly, Losh, Bellugi, & Wulfeck 2004).

4. Conclusion

The chapters in this volume discuss how research on language disorder can inform theories of language development. The body of work represented is impressive, and reviews a very large number of children with a variety of perceptual, cognitive and language disorders. While these children are experiencing difficulties, they are essentially learning their community language and not some bizarre version of it. While parts of their language systems may be compromised, there are remarkable strengths as well. The reader will be impressed with the breadth and depth of research on language disorder that has been conducted over the past 20 years. The outcome of the 2002 joint meeting of the IASCL and the SRCLD suggests a growing integration of research on the typical and atypical language development of children around the world.

Constraints on language development

Insights from developmental disorders

Michael S. C. Thomas

1. Introduction

When one assesses the language abilities of children and adults with developmental disorders, it is not uncommon to find an uneven profile across the sub-domains of language. Standardized tests for various aspects of language can exhibit a differential relationship compared both to each other and to overall (average) mental age (MA). For example, in a comparison of Down syndrome (DS), Williams syndrome (WS), autism and Fragile X (FraX), Fowler (1998) described dissociations between phonology, lexical semantics, morphosyntax and pragmatics. From these dissociations, it is evident that general cognition cannot be a reliable indicator of all aspects of language function in children with learning disabilities. While language acquisition typically lags behind MA-level expectations in children with learning disabilities, Fowler noted that disorders such as Williams syndrome and hydrocephalus with associated myelomeningocele appear superficially to be exceptions. From her comparison, Fowler concluded that pragmatics and lexical semantics are more closely tied to MA than phonology and morphosyntax.

Tager-Flusberg and Sullivan (1997) carried out a similar comparison of the same four disorders but this time seeking possible asynchronies in the early development of several areas of language semantic, grammatical, and pragmatic aspects. These authors also noted disparities in areas such as vocal development, social communicative development, gesture, lexical development, phonological development, early grammar and pragmatics.

However, despite the differences highlighted in their respective reviews, both Fowler (1998) and Tager-Flusberg and Sullivan (1997) also noted similarities across the disorders. For example in early development, there were consistent patterns of errors displayed in speech articulation; and in morphosyntax, although some disorders stopped short of mastery, the order of acquisition of syntactic structures appeared similar. In some senses, atypical language development generally retains some link with the normal profile of development.

What can this pattern of commonalities and dissociations tell us about the development of the language system? Two explanatory frameworks compete to interpret the results. One approach is based on the assumption of functional modularity in the normal adult system. The field of neuropsychology has identified case studies of healthy adults who exhibit selective deficits to different components of language following acquired brain damage. From these dissociations, a modular functional architecture has been inferred. Within modular theories, the linguistic performance of individuals with developmental language impairments is viewed as reflecting the architecture of the normal system but with selective components of this system under-developed or over-developed (Clahsen & Temple 2003). This framework provides a comfortable fit between the results of standardized language tests and atypical functional structure. Assuming we have tests that index the integrity of individual modules (e.g., tests of vocabulary, tests of grammar, tests of phonological awareness, and so on), scores in the normal range can be read off as reflecting a normally developed component and scores above or below the normal range can be read off as reflecting an (atypically) over- or under-developed component. This mapping of test results to modular structure in *developmental* disorders rests on one of two assumptions. Either the entire modular system identified in the adult is also present in the infant, so that language development can commence with an initial selective anomaly in one or more components; or the modular structure emerges to an extent through development, but in such a way that when things go wrong, some parts can emerge with atypical functionality while the rest manage to emerge with their normal functionality. Together, these alternatives constitute the assumption of *residual normality* (Thomas & Karmiloff-Smith 2002a). One further assumption is required for us to read off a normal score achieved on a standardized test as a guarantee of the normal functioning of an underlying component: that atypical cognitive processes could not generate the same normal score on this test.

The alternative framework, sometimes referred to as neuroconstructivism (Karmiloff-Smith 1998), places a much greater emphasis on the role of development in producing cognitive structure. It is based on the premise that the adult modular structure is not present in the infant but is itself a product of the developmental process. This is a view strongly motivated by data from developmental cognitive neuroscience (Elman, Bates, Johnson, Karmiloff-Smith, Parisi, & Plunkett 1996; Karmiloff-Smith 1998). This developmental perspective draws into question the sensitivity of standardized tests, raising the possibility that scores in the normal range may be achieved by atypical cognitive processes. Instead it is argued that sensitive on-line tasks are necessary to properly assess underlying processes (Karmiloff-Smith 1997; Karmiloff-Smith, Thomas, Annaz, Humphreys, Ewing, Grice, Brace, Van Duuren, Pike, & Campbell 2004). In the view of these authors, the clean pattern of normal versus impaired modules identified in some developmental disorders may in part be an artifact of the straightjacket of standardized tests. If a child takes a receptive vocabulary test, they can only possibly score below, at or above the normal range.

The debate between these two explanations of uneven linguistic profiles has at times become polarized. On the one hand, there are strong claims that for given developmental disorders, certain cognitive structures *must have* developed normally given behavior in the normal range (sometimes these are referred to as 'intact' or 'spared' systems). On the other hand there are counter claims that since the developmental processes we know about could not have produced such an uneven modular outcome, the relevant behavior *must be* produced by structures that are qualitatively different and atypical. For example, such polarization has occurred in evaluating syntax processing in Williams syndrome, and in evaluating the lexicon in the so-called 'grammatical' subtype of Specific Language Impairment.

Although my own previous work has been carried out within the neuroconstructivist framework, in this chapter my intention is to step back from this debate somewhat, and focus on exploring the notion of *constrained development*. This is because both frameworks must eventually incorporate an account of this sort, even if the strength of the constraints will differ in the two types of account. In the next section, I consider how both modular and neuroconstructivist frameworks still face significant challenges in characterizing the developmental process.

2. Development produces the disorder

In an older child, adolescent, or adult with a developmental language disorder, development has played some role in producing the observed behavioral deficits. The exact contribution of development is disputed. However, in both modular and neuroconstructivist frameworks, the nature of the developmental process remains obscure.

The modular approach de-emphasizes the contribution of development, placing the antecedents of deficits in particular components of a proto-language system already present in the infant. For example, various explanations of Specific Language Impairment (SLI) exist which propose a deficit restricted to abstract language structures involved in the rule-governed movement or combination of words into complex structures (see Ullman & Pierpont in press, for review). According to different versions, children may come to language impaired in their ability to establish structural relationships in sentences, such as agreement or specifier head-relations; or they may lack rules for linguistic features; or they may be stuck in a period of language development where marking of tense is taken to be optional; or they may be solely impaired on non-local dependency relations; or they may have problems with more general language functions such as learning implicit rules. Since the disorder is argued to have a strong genetic component, the implication is that such impairments pre-date acquisition.

Two aspects remain vague in the modular account. The first is the exact granularity of the proto-language system, that is, the miniature, content-free modular functional architecture present in the pre-linguistic infant (see Thomas & Karmiloff-Smith 2005, for discussion). The second is the developmental process by which this architecture acquires its content when exposed to a given social and linguistic environment. While some researchers argue there is scant empirical evidence for the existence of adult-like modular functional structure in the infant (e.g., Bates & Roe 2001; Elman et al. 1996), here we need merely point out that if one is going to argue for such a structure, one needs to say exactly what it looks like. At what level of detail do functional distinctions exist in the infant system – between sounds, meanings, motor actions, and social interactions; or between phonology, morphology, syntax, and the lexicon? Stipulating the granularity of the infant proto-system permits specification of the components may have initial developmental deficits. The account then needs to be complemented by specification of the processes of learning. Such processes must put particular content in each of the modular 'boxes' whilst allowing the components to interact fluidly in language comprehension and production. Even a strictly modular account of atypical language development needs to postulate a startstate (however constrained) and a pathway via a set of interactions with an information-laden world to deliver the final uneven structures observed in the adult developmental disorder.

While the neuroconstructivist approach accepts functional modularity as a possible characterization of the adult system, it rejects it as a startstate for the infant cognitive system. This approach rests on a theory that modularity emerges as a product of development, from a relatively less differentiated information processing system. The less differentiated system has capacities that are *relevant* to cognitive domains rather than specific to them (for instance, the ability of a mechanical to processes sequences may be relevant to syntax processing, without being specific to the linguistic structures that sentences contain). This initial flexibility is lost across development as the system commits its relevant capacities to particular domains. An explanation of developmental deficits consists in identifying how these initial domain relevancies have been altered in the disorder, and then how the subsequent process of emergent modularization has been perturbed (if indeed it has been). An emphasis on differences in the startstate leads neuroconstructivists to investigate the infant precursors of later uneven cognitive profiles (Karmiloff-Smith 1998). For example, Paterson, Brown, Gsödl, Johnson and Karmiloff-Smith (1999) noted that in adults with WS and DS, individuals with WS were relatively stronger than those with DS in language but the reverse was the case in the domain of number. When Paterson et al. explored the precursors of these cognitive skills in infants with the disorders, they found no advantage for toddlers with WS over DS in a language task, and *better* performance in WS than DS in the number task. The adult pattern was not replicated in the infant state, implying that different atypical developmental trajectories separate the populations (see Singer Harris, Bellugi, Bates, Jones, & Rossen 1997; Mervis & Robinson 2000, for discussion). These authors therefore argued against the idea that the atypical infant proto-cognitive system might contain a miniature version of the adult functional structure with the same pattern of strengths and weaknesses.

Two difficulties remain for the neuroconstructivist approach. The first difficulty is not unrelated to the one faced by the modular approach. Even if there are much weaker constraints on the startstate of the proto-language system, these still need to be identified. What is the set of initial domain-relevancies that pre-date language, and what is the nature of the process that eventually delivers domain-specific functional structures? The account eventually needs to be concrete enough to establish the strength of the constraints governing the emergence of modularity; what "seeds" does the proto-language system start with; what conditions would be sufficient to disrupt it; and how would a genuinely "atypical" functional structure behave. Presumably, even a system dealing in no more than domain relevancies must arrive with possible channels of information flow established – for example, between motor systems driving articulation, perceptual systems interpreting input, multi-modal systems linking to conceptual knowledge, and pragmatic systems linking with social and emotional systems. The second difficulty is that while neuroconstructivism prompts its adherents to build developmental trajectories from infancy through childhood to adult language structures, the empirical basis for "proto" cognitive structures is problematic. For example, Paterson et al. (1999) compared scores on receptive vocabulary tests in adults (i.e., selecting a picture that goes with a word from a set of alternatives) with performance on a preferential looking task in infants, where infants were presented with two pictures (e.g., a dog and a cat) and their gaze behavior monitored when they heard a label (e.g., "Look at the dog! Look at the dog!"). Where differences are found in the adult and infant pattern in a cross-syndrome comparison, how do we know that the two 'vocabulary' tasks are indexing the same mechanism? The problem even remains when the same task is used – how can we be sure that the same task is treated the same way at very different ages? We need to be able to rule out the possibility that data showing differential relative profiles in infancy and adulthood are not in fact the result of measuring different cognitive capacities at the two ages (such as, in the preceding example, lexical knowledge in the adult and attention/degree of novelty preference in the infant).

It is worth pointing out that evidence from brain imaging studies is often introduced in an attempt to distinguish modular and neuroconstructivist positions (predominantly by the latter group, as you may guess from the 'neuro' prefix). I won't discuss brain level evidence here, other than to suggest that it indicates that the effects of genetic mutations on brain development in developmental disorders tend to be widespread rather than focal (see Mareschal, Johnson, Sirios, Spratling, Thomas, & Westermann forthcoming; Karmiloff-Smith & Thomas 2003; Thomas 2003, for discussion); and that brain evidence has been interpreted both within modular and neuroconstructivist frameworks (e.g., for WS, see Reiss, Eckert, Rose, Karchemskiy, Kesler, Chang, Reynolds, Kwon, & Galaburda 2004; for a modular perspective; and for a neuroconstructivist perspective, Grice, Spratling, Karmiloff-Smith, Halit, Csibra, de Haan, & Johnson 2001; Karmiloff-Smith 1998; Neville, Mills, & Bellugi 1994; Mills, Alvarez, St. George, Appelbaum, Bellugi, & Neville 2000). Brain evidence remains problematic in that while it is suggestive, for instance in the lower degree of functional localization and specialization observed in the infant neocortex (Karmiloff-Smith 1998), it is not clear how brain function constrains the cognitive structures it is supporting at an given point in time (see Mareschal et al. forthcoming, for discussion).

Thus far, then, we have suggested that explanations of uneven language profiles are compromised by lack of an explicit developmental account of the origin of the architecture of the adult system. In the current chapter, I address this issue as follows. First I characterize some of the properties a developmental account should have with reference to the multiple components of the language system. Second, taking the example of Williams syndrome, I indicate the type of empirical evidence that might be used to identify the (atypical) constraints operating on development in a disorder. Third, I discuss some recent findings from computational modeling, a forum that permits a more precise exploration of the way in which atypical constraints on development could produce behavioral deficits in a given language domain.

3. Characterizing the developmental process

A cognitive-level developmental theory that explains the uneven language profile found in some disorders must emphasize three characteristics: *interactivity, compensation*, and *timing* (Thomas & Karmiloff-Smith 2005). In this section, I concentrate in the main on the first two of these (see Elman et al. 1996, for a more detailed consideration of timing).

3.1 Interactivity

Several authors have argued that early language development is characterized by *interactions* between multiple sources of information and the components that process them (e.g., Bishop 1997; Chiat 2001; Karmiloff-Smith 1997, 1998; McDonald 1997). For example, Chiat (2001) maintained that language acquisition should be construed as a mapping task between sound and meaning, through which the words and sentence structures of a language are established. To achieve this mapping, multiple sets of information are exploited. When semantics is ambiguous, phonology can be used to bootstrap the extraction of meaning. When phonology is ambiguous (for instance during lexical segmentation), semantics can be used to bootstrap the extraction of word-sound information. Together, phonological and semantic information help bootstrap the acquisition of morpho-syntax. In a developmental disorder where there are indications of differential deficits across the components of the language system, any explanation of behavioral impairments must incorporate the altered pattern of interactions (and their timing). Chiat (2001) carried out this exercise for SLI and favored an account that considers the language deficits in morphology and syntax as arising from impaired phonological processing. The phonological impairment then leads to consequent disruption of the interactions inherent in the mapping process.

A phonological account of SLI is consistent with the view that higher-level language deficits arise as a developmental consequence of lower level deficits, so that, for instance, the phonological impairments in SLI may themselves originate in low-level auditory processing problems. However, this theory is controversial in as much as some adults with SLI do not demonstrate low-level processing deficits in auditory discrimination (McArthur & Bishop 2004; Rosen 2003). One response is to postulate that auditory processing impairments may exist early in development and yet fail to be measurable in the mature system. This would be one instantiation of the claim that *timing* is an essential factor in producing developmental impairments. The failure to find an auditory processing deficit in an adult with SLI cannot be assumed to mean that such a processing deficit did not exist in infancy and make an impact on early language development. However, the postulation of unmeasurable causal factors is problematic. If one assumes that the source of an adult language problem lies in a cause that can no longer be measured, one might argue that the falsifiability of the low-level deficit theory is compromised. Of course, this simply highlights the point that developmental deficits demand that empirical data are collected across the course of development rather than just at its end-point. The early deficit theory is eminently testable using longitudinal studies in children with SLI or infants at risk for SLI.

The idea that low-level auditory processing deficits explain higher-level language problems in SLI is not supported as a *sufficient* condition by data comparing children with SLI and those with mild hearing impairments. Norbury, Bishop and Briscoe (2001) discovered phonological processing problems in both group but problems in productive inflectional morphology only in the SLI group. It appears that poor auditory processing is not necessarily associated with deficits in the more abstract, high-level aspects of language. In addition, even accepting the role of phonology, the causal pathway linking problems at this level to circumscribed syntactic difficulties (e.g., subject-verb number agreement) is at best obscure (though see Joanisse & Seidenberg 2003, for some preliminary attempts to make these links in the domain of anaphor resolution).

Nevertheless, at a broad level, the importance of the quality of language input has been emphasized by a comparative analysis carried out by McDonald (1997), which contrasted several typical and atypical populations that exhibited either successful or unsuccessful acquisition of language. These populations included late L2 learners, deaf sign-language learners, individuals with DS, individuals with WS and children with SLI. McDonald concluded that good representations of speech sounds were key in predicting the successful acquisition of a language including its syntax. Once again this supports the view that the components of the language system interact across development.

3.2 Compensation

The second characteristic that any theory of atypical language development must incorporate is *compensation*. The importance of compensation can be illustrated by a triangular comparison of adult aphasics, healthy children who have experienced early focal brain damage, and children with developmental disorders (see Karmiloff-Smith & Thomas 2003; Thomas 2003). The comparison goes as follows. (1) Following focal brain damage to their left hemispheres, adults can show persistent selective deficits in their language abilities (e.g., as exhibited in non-fluent and fluent aphasia). However, (2) following similar focal damage, healthy children usually then go on to demonstrate recovery from initial aphasic symptoms and later perform within the normal range on language tasks (see Bates & Roe 2001, for a review). Presumably, the greater effective plasticity of the child brain has permitted compensation and reorganization of function. As a consequence, when we (3) compare adults who had focal lesions when they were children with adults who have developmental disorders of language, we find significant deficits only in the latter. Of course, pointing to the presence of deficits in a developmental disorder is somewhat tautological, but the comparison nevertheless raises the question that if genetic developmental disorders of language are to be characterized by initial selective deficits to language-relevant structures, why has compensation-to-recovery not occurred as it does in the individuals experiencing early focal lesions? The answer is that compensation in the developmental disorder probably *has* occurred, but the constraints of the system are insufficient to allow performance to develop to a level within the normal range (Mareschal et al. forthcoming; Thomas 2003). This must be true for behaviorally defined disorders, because any child that had successfully compensated for their initial deficit would not be diagnosed as having a disorder. However there are parallels to be drawn between healthy children with early acquired brain damage and those with developmental disorders, but the relevant comparison is for healthy children who have experienced widespread and/or diffuse brain damage rather than focal lesions (see Thomas 2003).

Our account of the emergence of differentiated language structure in the adult will therefore need to incorporate interactivity, compensation, and timing, whether the early infant system is strongly or weakly constrained. This has significant implications for uneven profiles found in developmental disorders.

If we propose that the uneven profile can be explained by an initial deficit to a single component of the system (say, the proto-phonological system, proto-lexicon, proto-syntax system, or proto-pragmatic system), why wouldn't this impairment become smeared across other components through the interactions that occur between them during development? And why wouldn't other components in the system manage compensate for this selective deficit and so attenuate the impairment across development?

To take interactivity, if there were an initial selective impairment in pragmatics in infants with autism, one might expect the deficit to be passed to the lexicon, where words or phrases whose meaning can only be inferred from speaker intentions should not be acquired normally. One might expect non-canonical syntactic constructions (such as passives or cleft constructions) to be poorly processed, since these are predominantly employed in service of emphasizing the topic of the sentence for the listener, that is, for pragmatic reasons. To take compensation, if there were an initial selective impairment in syntax in SLI, why shouldn't the child compensate by using the lexicon to acquire common whole inflected forms and syntactic phrases, to be deployed in the appropriate communicative context and so avoid diagnosis as having a language impairment? The exact answers to these questions are not important in the current context (perhaps both phenomena occur; see Section 5 for further discussion of SLI). The point is that uneven language profiles may encourage the idea that selective damage has occurred, but explanations must be couched in terms of the development of differentiated language structures. If theories propose highly selective deficits in the adult with the disorder, then they must incorporate *developmental* reasons why neither interactivity nor compensation has taken place.

If one is to build an explanation of language deficits in terms of the developmental process, what type of empirical evidence should guide one's hand? In this next section, I use Williams syndrome as an illustration.

4. The example of Williams syndrome

Williams syndrome involves the deletion of some 25 genes from one of the copies of chromosome 7 (see Donnai & Karmiloff-Smith 2000, for full details of the syndrome). Individuals with WS usually present with IQs in the 50–60s range, with poor spatial and numerical cognition. While there is an initial delay in language development, by adolescence and adulthood many individuals display large vocabularies that co-exist with relatively good scores on standardized grammatical tests. Their language can include rich syntactic structure, with production and comprehension performance on complex syntactic structures (passives, relatives) in line with MA controls (Clahsen & Almazan 1998; Zukowski 2001).

In some respects, the developmental trajectory for language appears normal in WS. Thus, Mervis, Morris, Bertrand and Robinson (1999) noted that, while the syntactic abilities of children with WS (39 children from 2 years 6 months to 12 years of age) were considerably delayed, syntactic complexity was nonetheless appropriate for the mean length of utterance (MLU). This contrasts with DS, autism and FraX, where syntactic complexity turned out to be less than would be expected at MLUs over 3. This result prompted Mervis et al. to claim that WS is the first syndrome in which the normal relation between utterance length and complexity has been demonstrated. However, in other respects, the pattern is atypical. There are more errors in morphology (verb tense agreement, personal pronouns, grammatical gender; Karmiloff-Smith et al. 1997; Volterra, Capirci, Pezzini, Sabbadini, & Vicari 1996) than in syntax. Mervis et al. (1999) found that while the syntactic complexity scores of children with WS were significantly higher than would have been expected on the basis of spatial constructive ability, they were nevertheless significantly lower than would have been expected on the basis of receptive vocabulary ability, verbal ability, or auditory short-term memory. Across a large sample of 77 individuals between 5 and 52 years, Mervis et al. (1999) reported that performance on the Test of Receptive Grammar (Bishop 1983) was poor for complex constructions. Only 18% of the participants (22% of the adults) passed the test block that assessed relative clauses and only 5% (9% of the adults) passed the block assessing embedded sentences.

Such fractionation – patterns of strengths and weaknesses – appears in other areas of the WS language system (Thomas in press). Pragmatics, less advanced in WS than grammar, also exhibits within-domain fractionation. There is relatively good performance in social sensitivity (e.g., making dyadic eye contact, sensitivity to non-verbal cues) but problems in areas such as greeting behaviors, topic maintenance, and question answering (Semel & Rosner 2003). In lexical-semantics, a relative strength in category concepts (e.g., the distinction between animals, tools, clothing, furniture etc.) contrasts with problems understanding semantic relational concepts such as spatial-temporal terms (Phillips, Jarrold, Baddeley, Grant, & Karmiloff-Smith 2004). Even within category concepts, recent evidence has indicated differential naming problems across categories (Temple, Almazan, & Sherwood 2002; Thomas, Dockrell, Messer, Parmigiani, Ansari, & Karmiloff-Smith submitted), and it has been argued that the lexicon is an area with specific anomalies in WS (Clahsen & Almazan 1998; Rossen, Klima, Bellugi, Bihrle, & Jones 1996; Temple et al. 2002).

In order to consider the developmental origins of this uneven pattern, researchers have turned to precursors of language in WS infants. In Karmiloff-Smith and Thomas (2003), we recently reviewed this work. The most salient aspect of the onset of language in WS is that it is delayed. Although this delay is variable, one study of 54 children with WS found an average delay of 2 years, similar to that found for children with DS (Singer Harris et al. 1997; see also Paterson et al. 1999). Though delayed, some aspects of early development reveal normal behavioural patterns. For example, the onset of hand banging predicts the onset of canonical babbling in infants with WS in the same way as it does in typically developing infants (Masataka 2001; Mervis & Bertrand 1997).

Despite the fact that phonological memory appears as a relative strength in WS in childhood and adulthood (Mervis et al. 1999), a study of the ability of infants and toddlers with WS to segment the fluent speech stream into words revealed serious delays (Nazzi, Paterson, & Karmiloff-Smith 2003). In part, then, language delays may be due to problems with the early development of speech perception and phonological representations.

However, some precursors appear not just delayed but atypical. For example, Laing and colleagues examined socio-interactive precursors to language development in toddlers with WS compared with MA controls (Laing, Butterworth, Ansari, Gsödl, Longhi, Panagiotaki, Paterson, & Karmiloff-Smith 2002). Although toddlers with WS were proficient at dyadic interactions with a caregiver (and indeed sometimes exceeded the scores of MA controls due to persistent fixation on the caregiver's face; see also Bertrand, Mervis, Rice, & Adamson 1993; Jones, Bellugi, Lai, Chiles, Reilly, Lincoln, & Adolphs 2000), there was a marked deficiency in triadic interactions incorporating an object. Specifically, toddlers with WS had difficulty switching attention from the caregiver to an object that was being referred to in communication (via pointing, looking, and naming). Such a deficiency could disadvantage the toddlers with WS in learning the names of objects, since shared attention to newly named objects is one of the main routes into vocabulary acquisition. And indeed, there is accumulating evidence that precursors to vocabulary development in WS are atypical.

Typically developing infants use the presence of linguistic or gestural information that accompanies the introduction of novel objects to influence their subsequent categorisation of those objects, sometimes over and above the perceptual similarities among the objects. However, Nazzi and Karmiloff-Smith

(2002) found that 2- to 6-year-old children with WS were significantly less able than typical controls to use verbal cues to constrain categorisation. Masataka (2000) found a similar poverty in the ability of 2–3 year olds with WS to use gestural information to constrain categorisation.

In typically developing children, the ability to use pointing to refer to objects tends to emerge before the use of verbal labels for the same purpose. Presumably, pointing indexes the emergence of the cognitive ability to make reference, prior to the lexical manifestation. Pointing to objects and eliciting pointing behaviour in adults also facilitate the ability to find the correct referent for a given label. However, in WS, Mervis and Bertrand (1997) found that the order was reversed, with the onset of productive vocabulary *preceding* pointing. Laing et al. (2002) confirmed a deficit in the pointing behaviour of infants with WS, despite relative proficiency at fine motor skills. Vocabulary acquisition, therefore, appears to rely on a different set of cues and constraints in WS. When Stevens and Karmiloff-Smith (1997) examined the constraints that older children and young adults with WS were using to learn novel words, these, too, appeared atypical.

Relations between markers of semantic knowledge and productive vocabulary were also unusual in young children with WS. Spontaneous exhaustive sorting of objects (such as arranging toy animals and blocks into their separate categories) indexes the development of semantic knowledge and tends to precede a rapid rise in the rate of vocabulary acquisition in typically developing children. By the time children find it clear which categories objects fall into, it becomes increasingly easier for them to attach consistent labels to different objects. However, for children with WS, Mervis and Bertrand (1997) found no evidence that exhaustive sorting preceded the vocabulary spurt. Indeed, several children with WS exhibited the reverse pattern – unlike children with DS who always displayed the normal pattern.

Finally, there is preliminary evidence that compared to normal children the vocabulary of young children with WS exhibits a reduced advantage for comprehension vocabulary over production vocabulary (Paterson 2000), implying a relatively higher productive vocabulary for their level for comprehension.

In sum, the study of precursors to language development in WS reveals two main themes. First there is an overall delay, perhaps of a more generalized nature incorporating delays in at least motor, phonological, and semantic development. Second, when language development gets underway, a differential balance emerges between the ability to encode and produce word forms on the one hand, and the acquisition of the semantic underpinnings for those words on the other. However, characterization of the endstate language system in WS found in adolescents and adults remains controversial. Thomas and Karmiloff-Smith (2003) recently identified two main schools of theory. The first of these is more or less a null hypothesis. The *Conservative hypothesis* argues that the language we see in WS is not markedly atypical, just the product of delayed development combined with low IQ. The second school of theory develops the themes emerging from the study of early WS language development: the *Semantics-Phonology Imbalance hypothesis* comprises a cluster of claims that the WS language system involves a differential pattern of impairments across language.

The Conservative hypothesis runs as follows. Deficits in syntax and pragmatics in WS are what one might expect at a given level of mental retardation. Language development from the earliest age reflects the interests of a child with WS, specifically a strong desire for social interaction (e.g., Jones et al. 2000). Language is initially used more to mediate these interactions than as a referential tool. Subsequent vocabulary development reflects the special interests of the child with some degree of mental retardation, with unusual ('precocious') word usage employed as a strategic device to gain attention and mediate social interaction (Thomas et al. submitted). Deficits that do exist in vocabulary reflect other non-linguistic aspects of WS. For instance their visuo-spatial processing deficit leads to problems acquiring spatial vocabulary (Phillips, Jarrold, Baddeley, Grant, & Karmiloff-Smith 2004). The challenge for the Conservative hypothesis, however, is to explain why individuals with WS should show errors in, for instance, morphosyntax, that are not found in typically developing children, and why they should show predominantly successful language acquisition when individuals with other genetic syndromes involving mental retardation do not. To the latter point, one could respond that it is the other disorders that have the problems (say, in phonology, while in WS, after a delay, this develops within the normal range). Tager-Flusberg, Plesa-Skwerer, Faja and Joseph (2003: 10) provide a recent statement of the Conservative position: "Despite claims to the contrary... there is no evidence that children with WS acquire language any differently than other [typically developing] children, although they may be delayed in the onset of first words and phrases, as would be expected given their mental retardation."

By contrast, the Semantics-Phonology Imbalance hypothesis (really a cluster of related hypotheses) argues that language development in WS takes place under altered constraints. Several atypical constraints have been proposed. First, there is the idea that individuals with WS have a *particular strength in, or a sensitivity of, phonological short-term memory* (Majerus 2004; Majerus, Palmisano, van der Linden, Barisnikov, & Poncelet 2001; Mervis et al. 1999).

For example, Vicari, Carlesimo, Brizzolara and Pezzini (1996) have labeled language in WS as "hyper-phonological", and Bishop (1999) has argued that WS demonstrates the importance of short-term memory for speech sounds in determining the success of language development. Second, there is the proposal the WS exhibits *a particular weakness in lexical semantics*. Volterra and colleagues have noted that grammatical problems in WS are especially evident with those aspects of morphology carrying out a semantic function; and that individuals with WS perform better than mental-age match controls only in those areas of language where semantic aspects are not involved (e.g., Pezzini, Vicari, Volterra, Milani, & Ossella 1999; Volterra, Capirci, & Caselli 2001). Rossen et al. (1996) proposed that anomalous activation dynamics within the lexicon, specifically impaired inhibitory dynamics mediating context effects, lead to imprecise knowledge of concepts in WS and atypical vocabulary usage (see Temple et al. 2002, for a similar proposal; Thomas et al. submitted, for discussion). Third, there might be *a lag between the development of phonology and semantics* in WS, or a *problem integrating the two sources of information*. For example, Karmiloff-Smith, Tyler, Voice, Sims, Udwin, Howlin and Davies (1998) found that when individuals with WS monitored a sentence for a target word, performance was like controls in showing disruptions following syntactic violations. However there was a divergence when those violations involved lexically based information. Here the control group showed disruption of word monitoring, but the WS group did not. This led the authors to propose that in WS, there is a deficit in integrating lexical-semantic information with phonological information in real-time processing. Indeed, Frawley (2002) subsequently argued that WS language should be seen primarily as a disorder involving integration deficits between processing modules.

In all of these cases, the outcome of the imbalance is a system that relies (or has relied at certain points in its developmental history) more on phonological information than semantic information, with certain consequent behavioral impairments. A complication of the Imbalance theory is that most of its components are logically independent and not mutually exclusive. It is at least possible that several of the hypotheses could conjointly turn out to be true. For example, WS might constitute a case where there are differences in phonology and in semantics, in a system exhibiting general delay and overlying effects of mental retardation.

From the example of Williams syndrome, then, we can see an initial characterization of an uneven language profile in adolescence and adulthood, including claims that grammar has (selectively) developed normally (Clahsen & Almazan 1998). However, this initial modular proposal was not accompanied by any proposals for the developmental pathway (Thomas & Karmiloff-Smith 2005). Moreover, the characterization was tempered by the fact that even syntax development is delayed in WS and then does not reach normal levels of mastery. Subsequent testing has revealed a good deal of fractionation or unevenness of different aspects of WS language, including within syntax, the lexicon, and pragmatics. This raises questions of whether a modular account of WS language could possibly deal with the granularity of fractionation by postulating one or more deficits to the initial proto-language system. To do so would seem to require implausible levels of detailed structure in the infant prelinguistic system. The search for a developmental account then led to a focus on infant precursors, and here there accumulated evidence that some precursors to language were themselves atypical, for instance the deficit in triadic but not dyadic interaction, and the markers of referential communication. Although some researchers still prefer a "delayed but normal" explanation of WS language development, there is now a cluster of accounts that view this process in terms of an atypical balance between the lexical-semantic and phonological constraints, the former relatively weaker and the latter relatively stronger. In these accounts, the relatively high level of syntactic performance would be associated with the basis of good (albeit delayed) phonology. However, discussions still persist concerning whether syntax development itself follows a 'normal' course, and if it does, what this tells us of the constraints guiding typical and atypical language acquisition.

5. Computational investigations into constrained development

The methodology of computational modeling forms a convergent approach to understanding constraints on development, and how atypical constraints may produce sub-optimal development. Computational models provides a concrete basis to investigate more precisely how sources of information interact in the acquisition of a particular language domain, including opportunities for compensation, and the different ways in which delay and deviation may emerge from a system learning a facet of language. As with all methodologies, there are some limitations. Modeling necessarily involves simplification, and thus far it has focused in the main on individual domains (lexical segmentation, vocabulary acquisition, inflectional morphology, syntax processing; see Christiansen & Chater 2001) rather than the development and operation of multi-component systems (see Thomas & Karmiloff-Smith 2002a; Thomas &

Richardson in press, for discussion). Nevertheless, work to date has generated insights into the potential causes of developmental language deficits.

One of the main modeling formats applied to developmental disorders has been that of connectionist networks (see Thomas & Karmiloff-Smith 2002b, for a review). These are advantageous because the networks of simple processing units are learning systems that can acquire the structure of cognitive domains through training. Additionally, they contain computational parameters that alter the efficiency of learning, and so provide a tool to explore non-optimal conditions for acquisition. In the following paragraphs, I discuss four different theoretical issues I and various colleagues have investigated using connectionist modeling.

5.1 The contribution of the developmental process to producing behavioral impairments

In one model, we explored the implications of damaging a learning system in its initial state (analogous to a developmental disorder) compared to damaging a system in its trained state (analogous to an adult acquired deficit) as a way of gauging the potential contribution of a developmental process to generating behavioral impairments (Thomas & Karmiloff-Smith 2002a). The results demonstrated that some types of damage hurt an information processing system much more in its 'adult' state (e.g., severing network connections) while others hurt the system much more in the 'infant' state (e.g., adding noise to processing or blurring the input). The adult system can tolerate noise because it already has an accurate representation of the knowledge, but loss of network structure leads to a decrement in performance since connections contain established knowledge. By contrast, the infant system can tolerate loss of connections because it can organize remaining resources to acquire the knowledge, but the infant system is impaired by noisy processing because this blurs the knowledge that has to be acquired. This result echoes the conclusion of McDonald (1997) that a key factor in predicting the success of language acquisition across typical and atypical populations is whether the child has good representations of speech sounds.

5.2 Case study: English past tense formation in Williams syndrome

In other work, we have applied connectionist models to a much more detailed, data-driven consideration of one domain and one developmental disorder, the acquisition of English past tense formation in Williams syndrome (Thomas

& Karmiloff-Smith 2003). The model combines lexical-semantic information about a verb with phonological information about the verb's stem to generate its past tense form (Thomas & Karmiloff-Smith 2003; see Lavric, Pizzagalli, Forstmeier, & Rippon 2001 for discussion of this architecture). It thus allows detailed consideration of the relative influence of lexical-semantic and phonological constraints on the acquisition of this aspect of morphosyntax. As an outcome of the *normal* developmental process, the network comes to rely differentially on the two sources of information for driving two types of inflection, regular past tenses (talk ⇒ talked, wug ⇒ wugged) and irregular past tenses (go ⇒ went, hit ⇒ hit, think ⇒ thought). In particular, the system relies more heavily on lexical-semantic information for driving irregular inflections, so that in the trained model, a lesion to lexical-semantics differentially impairs irregulars (see also Joanisse & Seidenberg 1999). Our simulations focused on a cross-sectional developmental trajectory for the acquisition of regular, irregular, and novel verb past tense formation that we had generated from around 20 individuals with WS and 50 control children and adults (Thomas et al. 2001). These data indicated that individuals with WS exhibited a delay in the acquisition of the English past tense that was equal for regular and irregular verbs, but also a reduced tendency to generalize known inflectional patterns to novel verb forms.

We then set out to explore whether alterations to the model's initial constraints could account for these three features of the WS data. As we have seen, various claims have been made that there are subtle differences in the language system of individuals with Williams syndrome, including the proposals that their phonological representations may be atypical and perhaps rely on sensitive auditory processing, that their semantic representations may be atypical, or that semantic information about words may integrate poorly with phonology. Having established that the model could capture the normal developmental trajectory in this domain, we altered the initial constraints of the untrained network model to implement each type of proposed deficit. The results revealed that a manipulation of the phonological representations that reduced their similarity and redundancy was sufficient to reproduce the delay for regular and irregular past tense forms, as well as the reduction in generalization. Second, the pattern could also be produced when noise was added to the information coming from the semantic system during the acquisition of the past tense. Third, elimination or weakening of the semantic contribution produced a pattern inconsistent with this set of WS data comprising a selective delay for irregular verbs and no reduction in generalization (though see Clahsen & Almazan 1998, for a report of this pattern in a small sample of

4 children with WS). Lastly, slowed learning failed to produce a reduction in generalization, suggesting that delayed development alone was insufficient to explain WS performance and that atypical computational constraints are likely to be involved. This detailed modeling work was therefore able to test the viability of several competing hypotheses on the causes of particular language impairments in Williams syndrome. Manipulations to phonology or to the integration of phonology and semantics were able to simulate the past tense data; manipulations to semantics alone or delayed development were not.

5.3 Domain-specific versus domain-general deficits: A possible approach to explaining behavioral impairments in SLI

In a wider exploration of the model described above, we found that altering a 'domain-general' internal computational constraint prior to exposure to the problem domain could change the network's balance between the way it exploited lexical-semantic and phonological information during learning (Thomas in press). With this atypical parameter setting, the network generated a profile of performance on English past tense acquisition that is not dissimilar to that reported for children with SLI. For example, van der Lely and Ullman (2001) reported that in a past tense elicitation task, children with SLI showed low levels of inflection for both regular and irregular verbs (10–20% correct) and similarly low levels of extension of the regular rule to novel stems. Since regulars are normally inflected more accurately than irregulars, this amounts to a greater deficit for regular verbs – one might view this as a kind of developmental fractionation. Van der Lely and Ullman's explanation of this pattern of behavior relies on a linguistic theory that distinguishes separate mechanisms for acquiring regular and irregular verbs (Pinker 1991). Regulars are learned by a rule-implementing mechanism whereas irregulars are learned by an associative memory (see Ullman & Pierpont 2005, for a similar account where the two mechanisms are aligned with procedural and declarative memory systems in the brain). According to Ullman and colleagues, the children with SLI are unable to learn the regular rule due to an initial impairment in their rule-based/procedural system and the few regulars and irregulars that are correctly inflected reflect the compensatory action of the associative/declarative system. The idea that regulars are now inflected by a compensating associative memory system instead of a rule mechanism in the SLI group is supported by evidence of abnormally large frequency effects for regular verbs – frequency effects are taken to be the hallmark of domain-general associative memory.

It is important to be clear about the chain of inference in this case, because it clearly illustrates how researchers can move from behavioral evidence to deducing structural fractionations of the language system. The relatively greater impairment of regular inflections, along with the increased frequency effects in residual regular inflection are taken as evidence that in SLI, there has been a startstate deficit to a *domain-specific* computational structure responsible for learning regular past tense forms. It is important because the connectionist past tense model was able to simulate the same behavioral data without postulating any domain-specific fractionation, and moreover, exhibit the behavioral pattern as the product of an implemented developmental process.

To understand how the model simulated these data, we need to understand a little more about it. The model employs a 'three-layer' architecture, where a layer of internal processing units intercedes between the input layer (in this case representing lexical-semantics and verb-stem phonology) and the output layer (here representing inflected verb phonology). This internal or hidden layer is a common representational resource involved in processing regular, irregular, and novel inflections. The manipulation we applied to the network was to alter the initial properties of these hidden layer units. In particular, we reduced the sharpness of their thresholding functions. This manipulation roughly had the effect of attenuating the 'discriminability' of the units, making all computations fuzzier. The network was less able to learn sharp category boundaries in the problem domain to which it was exposed, requiring far more training than normal to generate these discriminations.

When the disordered network was 'aged-matched' to a normally developing past tense network, it exhibited low levels of regular and irregular inflection, along with poor regularization of novel stems. In other words, the disordered network gave an approximate fit to the SLI data presented by van der Lely and Ullman (2001). Importantly, in the model just as in the empirical data, regular verbs now exhibited an elevated frequency effect. Subsequent analysis of the network revealed that this was because regular inflection was being driven more strongly by lexical-semantic input than in the normal network. In effect, the system was treating regulars in the same way as irregulars, as if all verbs were exceptions to be generated via support from the lexicon.

On the face of it, this model would appear to parallel van der Lely and Ullman's explanation of their SLI data: residual regular inflection reflects the action of the declarative memory system storing word-specific information. Similarly, regulars and irregulars were treated in the same way in the disordered network, with equivalent reliance of lexical-semantics and equivalent sized frequency effects. Crucially, however, the startstate manipulation to the connectionist network was not to a domain-specific processing structure affecting only regulars, as assumed by Ullman and Pierpont and van der Lely. Instead, the computational manipulation targeted a general processing resource used to inflect both regular and irregular verbs. However, the particular computational property altered was one upon which regular verbs differentially relied. Regular verbs differ yet must all be treated in the same way. This requires sharp category boundaries that delineate regular space in which all items will be treated the same. The ability to learn sharp category boundaries might be seen as a computational property that is *relevant* to the domain of regular part of tense formation. The alteration of this domain-relevant property resulted in a deflection of the developmental trajectory such that, in terms of the relative size of deficits, there was an apparent fractionation between regular and irregular verbs. These initial alterations to the common computational resource additionally had the effect of altering the balance of the information sources on which the network relied to generate past tense forms. Phonological regularities were downplayed, while word-specific information was emphasized. The atypical constraints of the learning system served to alter the interaction between phonological and semantic sources of knowledge during development of this morpho-syntactic ability.

In sum, this modeling result demonstrates that behavioral evidence taken by van der Lely and Ullman (2001) and Ullman and Pierpont (in press) to indicate a structural fractionation of the language system in SLI could also be explained in terms of a learning system without such a fractionation, and the initial manipulation of a computational parameter with no specific reference to regular or irregular verbs.

5.4 Inferences from the comparison of developmental profiles across disorders

Modeling work also sheds light on the interpretation of similarities and differences in the way different disorder groups acquire language. The fact that we can take a model of normal development and create developmentally impaired systems of various types (noisy systems, systems with memory impairments, slow learners, and so on) allows us to explore the extent to which qualitatively different behavioral profiles are generated by altered internal constraints. We explored this in two recent models: the past tense model already discussed and a model of syntax acquisition.

One explanation of the similarities identified between the developmental profiles and patterns of errors across different disorders is that these similarities reflect immovable internal constraints of the language learning system (Newport 1990). The notion of a 'developmental delay' is predicated on identifying such similarities in children who do not reach the landmarks at the correct ages. It is deployed even in the case where mastery is never reached. Similarities may therefore be taken to imply that nothing is qualitatively different in the system: it is just not 'working very well'. However, it is also possible that similarities between typical and atypical development have another explanation: the range of behaviors that individuals can exhibit in language development is constrained by the common physical, social, and informational environment in which each individual's cognitive system is embedded. More specifically, behaviors normal or otherwise are in part constrained by the structure of the problem domain to which the cognitive system is exposed, whatever its underlying architecture. The extent to which cognitive architecture is *visible* in the behavioral changes and error patterns exhibited across development is a serious and unresolved issue. The simplest illustration of this idea is a cognitive domain that has an easy part and a hard part. A wide range of learning systems would naturally acquire the easy part before the hard part. Consequently, a common developmental profile here would tell us little about the actual learning system involved. To investigate this proposal, we exposed a variety of associative architectures to the past tense domain, varying the computational resources that the learning system brought to the problem (Mareschal et al. forthcoming). The results indicated that there was indeed great variation across the developmental profiles. However, the systems also exhibited similarities in their profiles. In particular, regular verb acquisition was usually in advance of irregular acquisition, and generalization of the regular rule was usually weaker to novel stems that rhymed with irregulars than to those that did not. These patterns were a result of the structure of common past tense domain that each model learned, including the similarities between verbs and type and token frequencies of the various items involved.

Dick et al. (2001, 2004) recently argued that similarities in syntactic deficits found in adults with aphasia and in children with developmental language impairments can also be traced to features of the shared problem domain. In particular, in a comprehension task (agent-patient role assignment), low frequency constructions and non-canonical subject-object word order constructions such as passives and object clefts ('the cat was chased by the dog', 'it was the cat that the dog chased') revealed greater behavioral impairments than high frequency and canonical order constructions like actives and subject clefts ('the dog chased the cat', 'it was the dog that chased the cat'). We trained a recurrent, sequence processing connectionist network on sentences of this form in the frequency that young children hear them (Thomas & Redington 2004). The network had to perform the same comprehension task as human subjects, identifying the agent in each sentence. The trained network showed the normal adult pattern of difficulty across the constructions. When it was trained with an initially reduced level of computational resources, it was also successful in simulating the exaggerated pattern of difficulty shown by children with developmental disorders. Importantly, the model also demonstrated relatively less vulnerability of constructions learned on the basis of unique lexical cues (such as passives, indicated by the word 'by') and relatively more vulnerability of constructions learned on the basis of sequence cues (such as object clefts, indicated by the two nouns that are not split by an intervening verb). The behavioral data (Dick et al. 2004) were also consistent with this differential effect. This pattern emerges in the model because reducing the initial computational resources produces a greater impairment in analyzing global information across sentences than in analyzing local information from individual lexical items. The consequence is that although the structure of the task domain paints a broad picture of task difficulty, the strengths and weaknesses of the computational learning system modulate this pattern.

In sum, models of two different aspects of grammar acquisition demonstrate that some similarities between atypical and normal development are the consequence of the problem domain. Disordered learning systems only serve to modify this pattern, sometimes in subtle ways. This line of computational work indicates firstly that the attributions of language disorders to 'developmental delay' on the basis of an absence of 'qualitative' differences need to be treated with caution; and secondly, the inference that behavioral similarities across different populations reflect internal constraints is not a secure one – they may as easily reflect external constraints.

6. Conclusions

In this chapter, we have considered how atypical profiles of language impairments may be informative about language acquisition. I have argued that the appropriate framework for explanations of deficits in developmental disorders is in terms of constraints on the developmental process – whether a given theory assumes the presence of domain-specific modular structure prior to language acquisition or assumes that such structure is the product of the developmental process itself. We considered characteristics that the atypical developmental process should incorporate such as interactivity and compensation.

If these characteristics do not figure within the developmental process, theories must explicitly stipulate why they should not occur. The example of Williams syndrome was used to illustrate how researchers can begin to identify the particular constraints that have deflected language development in an atypical population. Finally, computational modeling of atypical language acquisition was discussed, both as a method for testing whether a given set of atypical constraints (such as the balance of phonological and lexical-semantic information) is sufficient to generate particular behavioral impairments, and also as a way to assess the strength of inferences drawn from behavioral data. In the case of the latter, we saw how modeling indicated that behavioral dissociations in language development do not necessarily imply underlying structural fractionations, and how behavioral similarities between typical and atypical language acquisition do not necessarily stem from shared internal constraints but from the structure of the problem domain. Finally, we must note the context of this research. Understanding the constraints that shape and deflect the acquisition of language is an important step towards understanding how we may intervene to optimize the outcome of language learning in atypical populations.

Constructions and language development

Implications for language impairment

Paul Fletcher, Stephanie Stokes and Anita Wong

1. Introduction

Since the 1970s, the study of the grammatical progress of typically developing pre-school children has been of central importance for the investigation and assessment of children with language impairment. Over the three decades of the modern history of language acquisition studies, however, theoretical perspectives on grammatical development have changed considerably. Here we review those developments historically, and consider their implications for the investigation of language impairment, with particular attention to Cantonese. In particular we consider the potential effect on the study of language impairment of constructionist approaches to language development. If acquiring syntax is not what we think, as Tomasello (2000a) asserts, how would or should the reconceptualization he advocates impact on the way we evaluate and manage individuals with language impairment?

2. The historical background

The 1970s saw the burgeoning of interest in language acquisition studies. This was driven theoretically by Chomskyan linguistics, and empirically by the method and results of Roger Brown's project at Harvard focusing on the development of three children. The first fruits of this are summarized in Brown (1973). However the work of Brown's collaborators, and a new lease of life given to the data from Adam, Eve and Sarah by its publication in the CHILDES database have given the project contemporary influence in studies of typically developing children. This can be seen in the continuing popularity of longitudinal studies, and especially in the centrality of grammar in the analysis of children's progress. Brown (1973) concentrated in his detailed exposition on early semantic roles and grammatical relations, and on morphosyntax. Grammar, in various guises, continues to be the lens of choice through which language development is scrutinized. This has also been true of the study of atypical development, over a similar time span. Shortly after the publication of Brown's major work on language development, we find in Morehead and Morehead (1976) papers which address the grammatical abilities of individuals with language impairment. In one of them Johnston and Schery (1976) examined the same set of fourteen English morphemes that Brown had investigated. They found that children with language impairment acquired these forms in the same order as typically developing children, but at later language levels (as measured by MLU) and greater ages. In another paper in the same volume, Morehead and Ingram (1976) similarly used Brown's linguistic levels as defined by MLU to identify language status in groups of children developing typically and atypically, and examined their phrase structure and transformational rule systems. (The grammatical framework within which they were working was that of Chomsky 1965). Their general conclusion is that:

> ...the major differences between normal and linguistically deviant children of comparable linguistic level were not in the organization or occurrence of specific components of their base syntactic systems. Rather the significant differences were found in the onset and acquisition time necessary for learning base syntax and the use of aspects of that system, once acquired, for producing major lexical items in a variety of utterances.
>
> (Morehead & Ingram 1976: 223–224)

This finding confirms Johnston and Schery's conclusion that while the acquisition of grammar on the part of children with impairment might be delayed, even very delayed, it follows much the same course as development in typically developing children. This has been a guiding principle for studies of language impairment ever since. Initially it led to the construction of assessment procedures for clinical use which were based on the trajectory of typical grammatical development emerging from studies such as that of Brown (1973). Thus Crystal, Fletcher and Garman (1976) developed LARSP, a Language Assessment, Remediation and Screening Procedure. This was designed to identify grammatical categories and constructions used by the child in a sample of speech. LARSP used the descriptive framework of Quirk, Greenbaum, Leech and Svartvik (1972), to order phrasal and clausal constructions of increasing complexity in a series of stages. Location of the grammar of a child under review to a particular stage would inform the clinician's selection of target constructions for intervention. (See also Miller 1981 for a procedure with similar principles but using a different grammatical framework.)

The grammar-centered clinical assessments such as LARSP certainly facilitated a systematic approach to the characterization of the child's current state of grammatical knowledge. This in itself was an advance for clinical practice. But the procedures had inherent limitations. In part these were built in to the grammatical frameworks on which they were based. But more significant was their lack of attention to the lexicon. The 'flight to abstraction' built in to a grammatically-based description essentially ignores the lexical instantiation of grammatical categories. The assignment of a clausal label such as SVO to a child's utterance, or Det Adj N to part of it, omits from the record the lexical dimension of the child's language use, even though this is an integral part of her knowledge of the language. The significance of lexical organization in grammar has broadened considerably as Chomskyan theory has evolved. And in constructional approaches (e.g. Goldberg 1995; Tomasello 2003), we find the lexical instantiation of syntactic structures playing a central role. In what follows we will trace the increasing importance of the lexicon in grammatical theory, evaluate the relevance of a lexical perspective for tracking language impairment in Cantonese, and consider more generally the implications of an enhanced lexical perspective for the study of language impairment.

3. The lexicon in grammar

3.1 The developing role of the lexicon in grammar

In Chomsky's (1957) earliest formulation of a transformational grammar, the structure of the lexicon reflected the Bloomfieldian view that it was here that the irreducible irregularity of the language resided. Grammars are to a certain extent amenable to generalizations and rule statements, but there are limits. Beyond these limits we simply have to rely on lists of nouns, or verbs, or other categories. In Chomsky (1957) the lexicon is a separate component of the grammar (the others being phrase structure rules and transformations) which provides lists of words under category headings such as N, V, Adj, Modal. The implication is of very limited lexical structure beyond category membership, with lexical items made available for insertion under the terminal (category) nodes of the phrase structure tree. By the time of the Aspects model (Chomsky 1965), considerably more information relevant to syntax was incorporated into the lexicon. Lexical entries for major category items now included subcategorization information. So the entry for a verb, for example, would include as well as its category feature, its syntactic context in terms of obligatory and optional arguments. Thus optionally transitive verbs such as *move* could be distinguished from true intransitives such as *laugh* by the availability for the former of an optional NP argument. Later formulations augment the role of the lexicon further. Webelhuth (1995) points out that in the Government and Binding framework, the availability of detailed lexical entries, plus the projection principle could 'reduce language-particular base components to the setting of a few simple X-bar-theoretic parameters' (Webelhuth 1995: 34). The projection principle ensures that at all syntactic levels of representation, lexical items appear only in the contexts specified in their lexical entries. Trask (1993: 159) notes the growing importance of the lexicon, and sees it as 'one of the most striking trends in syntax'. The greater share of responsibility borne by the lexicon in grammatical theory over the period from the mid-1970s to the mid-1990s is reflected mainly in the interest shown in verb argument structure acquisition in typically developing children, from Pinker (1989) on. Some attention has also been paid to this issue in children with language impairment (see for example Chiat; 2003, Ingham, Fletcher, Schelletter, & Sinka 1998; O'Hara & Johnston 1997).

3.2 Construction grammar

Within the continuing development of Chomskyan grammars, then, the roles and responsibilities of the components of the grammar change. But even if there is now assumed to be more extensive coverage of grammar within the lexicon, a line is still drawn between components – between the lexicon and the 'computational core' of the grammar. An alternative approach, labeled construction grammar, erases this distinction and, it is argued, provides a more tractable framework for characterizing language development (Tomasello 1998). By extension, and maintaining the assumption of comparability between the trajectories of typical and atypical development, this framework may also be suited to the investigation of language impairment.

The constructional approach does not draw a line at some arbitrary point between lexis and syntax, but accepts a continuum between the two:

> Constructions can be thought of as the same theoretical type of representation object as lexical items, albeit syntactically complex and at least partially

> schematic. There is a CONTINUUM between the lexicon and syntactic constructions. (Croft 2001: 16–17)

This perspective is exploited in describing language development first of all by emphasising the similarity between learning words and learning grammar. In responding to the input they hear, children in the early stages of language development, around two years of age, may have in their repertoires a range of items of varying types, ranging from individual words through some morphemes to stereotyped greetings phrases to constructions of limited productivity based on learned sequences such as *Where's the X*. What we see here, in this view, is not a sequence of language development which proceeds from word-learning to the combining of these words according to syntactic rules they have learned. Rather:

> children learn simultaneously from adult utterances meaningful linguistic structures of many shapes and sizes and degrees of abstraction, and they then produce their own utterances on particular occasions of use by piecing together some of these many and variegated units in ways that express their immediate communicative intention. (Tomasello 2003: 99–100)

On this view we would expect to find, especially at the early stages of a child's learning of a language, a relatively unorganised system, even though there are several instances in the child's speech of past tense marking, prepositions and transitive sentences. In relation to the latter, the evidence suggests that for children under three, the transitivity of these sentences is specific to the verbs which appear in them. Initially, what would within a LARSP analysis system be labelled SVO sentences do not yet deserve such an abstract label, but instead are item-based constructions which rely on the child's knowledge of specific verbs. Tomasello (2003) provides evidence from both spontaneous speech and experimental studies to buttress this claim. If the claim holds for the early typically developing children, it has immediate relevance for children with language impairment. Tomasello (2000b) reviews a number of studies in which typically developing children were required to generalise a novel verb to use in a SVO sentence after hearing it used in another syntactic context. The results indicate that use of novel verbs in SVO sentences only becomes productive during the third and fourth years of life. That is, an abstract SVO construction is a relatively late development. Since many studies which have compared children with specific language impairment (SLI) and language-matched controls have found an age discrepancy of at least two years between the groups (see for example Wong, Leonard, Fletcher, & Stokes 2004), this suggests that school-age children with SLI may still be operating with item-based constructions for transitivity. In requiring us to consider lexis and syntax together, and in requiring detailed consideration of progress towards abstraction, rather than assuming it from the outset, the constructional approach has consequences for our study of SLI. These involve how we evaluate the language of children with SLI, how we identify intervention targets, and how we structure intervention itself. We will return to these general issues after considering the possible relevance of the constructional approach to the language of Cantonese-speaking children with SLI.

4. Specific language impairment in Cantonese

4.1 The characteristics of Cantonese

Cantonese is a language spoken in the southern Chinese province of Guangdong, in Hong Kong, and widely around the world wherever the Chinese diaspora took inhabitants from this region. As a Sino-Tibetan language with typical isolating characteristics, Cantonese has lexical items that are unvarying in form. There are no morphological paradigms for lexical categories. Indeed, the morphosyntactic processes that have been the focus of much of the work on the grammatical symptoms of language impairment in European languages are irrelevant for Cantonese. Verb tense and agreement, noun phrase agreement, or the effects of finiteness on constituent order (e.g. verb second requirements for finite forms in German), do not apply in Cantonese. There are temporal morphemes that post-modify verbs, notably a set of six aspect markers (Matthews & Yip 1994: 198ff.), but these are optional. Consequently, unlike English, Cantonese has no obligatory morphosyntactic elements available for scrutiny, and elements of the tense/agreement/copula complex are unavailable as phenotypic markers for SLI. The basic constituent order is SVO, but arguments can be fronted for topic prominence. Cantonese is a discourse-oriented language – verb arguments can be omitted from utterances when their referents are identifiable from the linguistic or non-linguistic context.

It is not possible to tell in advance whether a hitherto unstudied language is likely to present fewer acquisitional challenges to a learner, or simply different challenges to those we have become accustomed to seeing in English (Johnston 2004). In one area, that of segmentation, the identification of the boundaries of lexical and grammatical items should be more straightforward than it is in English, for example. Cantonese, like its Sinitic counterparts is a tonal language. Lexical and grammatical forms carry one of six contrastive tones. Lexical forms can consist of one or more syllables; grammatical morphemes tend to be single syllables. The language has a relatively simple syllable structure, which can be summarized as (C)V(V)(C). There are nineteen possible initial consonants, but only two sets of consonants – six items in all – can appear at the end of syllables: one of three nasals, and unreleased -p, -t, -k (Bauer & Benedict 1997). The fact that every syllable has to have a tone, and the asymmetry of consonant systems in initial and final position, suggest that Cantonese should be a relatively easy language for learners to segment syllabically (Peters 1997: 140). The placement of a contrastive tone on each syllable, whether it represents a lexical or grammatical morpheme, implies also that there will be no prosodic difference between members of lexical and grammatical categories. There is none of the phonetic erosion that characterizes verb forms in English for example, where stress reduction and other factors reduce the phonetic salience for these forms This has been argued to play a role in their learnability (Gleitman & Wanner 1982), or to render them vulnerable in the speech of children with SLI, under the demands of real-time processing (Leonard 2000: 125).

The relative ease of identification of morpheme boundaries may however be balanced by greater difficulties elsewhere. The discourse-oriented character of Cantonese means that in many situations where the information can be inferred from discourse, the marker of the aspectual nature of an event, or an argument identifying the direct or indirect object of a verb, will not be overtly present in an utterance. This 'optionality' of constituents, and the resulting variation in language models presented to the child, could present difficulties for a learner (Stokes 2002).

4.2 Specific language impairment in Cantonese

The definition of SLI requires observably intact neurological and hearing status, and normal intelligence and behavioral status. The initial diagnosis also requires performance on standardized language tests that is below some criterion, most often minus 1.25 standard deviations. By making use of available tests in Hong Kong, we have determined that it is possible to use these criteria to locate a group of Cantonese-speaking impaired children. Separate studies in Hong Kong have now identified groups of children with SLI. In one group of 60 children referred by Child Assessment Centres as potentially SLI, 26 turned out to meet the criteria. Half of these children were receptively and expressively delayed, and half were expressively delayed. The 24 children who could not be included in an SLI sample either did not complete testing, did not meet exclusion criteria, or failed to meet inclusion criteria on standardized language tests

(Stokes & Fletcher 2000). In a second study, 14 children were studied longitudinally for two years (Wong, Stokes & Fletcher 2003). And in a cross-sectional study comparing children with SLI with children matched for chronological age and with a group of younger typically developing children, 15 impaired individuals have been identified (Wong et al. 2004).

4.3 Faultlines in the language of Cantonese-speaking children with language impairment (CSLI)

4.3.1 *The implications of limited lexical diversity*

The implications of a constructional grammar approach to the characterisation of language impairment are far-reaching. For example, if the road to abstraction is long, as in the case of transitivity (Tomasello 2000b), and typically-developing children only generalise transitive relations in their third to fourth year, we would predict that children with SLI would arrive late at this destination, among others. Indirect indications that this is the case arise from studies of lexis in Cantonese-speaking children with SLI.

In arriving at a metric for lexical diversity in the speech of typically and atypically developing children, researchers have used various kinds of type-token ratios (e.g. Miller 1981), or they have computed the number of different words (NDW) occurring in a sample controlled for number of utterances (Miller 1991) or words (Klee 1992). More recently, in an attempt to avoid the problems associated with existing measures, Malvern, Richards, Chipere and Duran (2004), have developed a new measure, D. In an application of this measure to Cantonese-speaking children, Klee, Stokes, Wong, Fletcher and Gavin (2004) found that it discriminated a group of children with SLI from their age peers. They also found that D and MLU, together with age, could be used to distinguish the children with SLI from their language matched peers (a group of children on average two years younger than the children with SLI). The findings indicate that the children with SLI produce utterances with significantly less diverse vocabularies than their unaffected age peers, and that their reduced lexical abilities play a role in differentiating their performance from that of younger typically developing children.

Since D is arrived at by repeated sampling of all words in a transcript, it can only point to a general lexical deficiency (or advantage) in a child or group of children. Also, the study by Klee et al. (2004) is cross-sectional. To address the potential integration of lexis and grammar more directly, in relation to SVO constructions, we need a more specific examination of verb diversity. And generally, in order to map the path towards constructions in children whether they

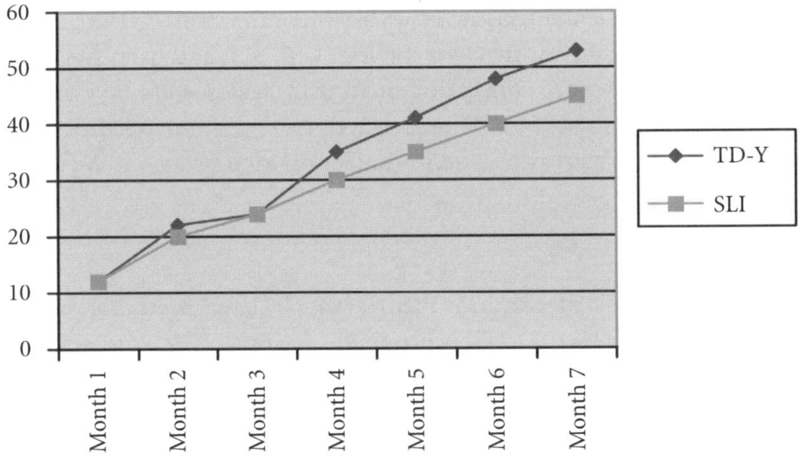

Figure 1. Use of new verbs over time by SLI and TD-Y groups

are developing typically or atypically, we need longitudinal information. While databases that follow children's development over time are relatively common for typical development, they are vanishingly rare in studies of SLI (though see Rice 2004 for an example for English). However Stokes, Fletcher and Leung (1997) followed a group of Cantonese-speaking children with SLI over a two year period, and data on their use of verbs indicates differences between them and a younger typically developing group.

The two groups (henceforth SLI and TD-Y) were matched for MLU at the outset of the study, and their use of transitive verbs was monitored at monthly intervals for the first seven months of the study. At the outset the average age of the SLI group was 53 months, and of the TD-Y group 36 months. Figure 1 shows the cumulative 'new transitive verb' total for each month over this period. Monthly gains in verbs were computed on the basis of verb types that had not appeared in the previous month's sample. The new verb total was then added to the verb total for the previous month to give total number of verb types. Verb tokens were held constant. As Figure 1 shows, by the end of a seven month period, the SLI group deploys around 20% fewer verbs than the TD-Y group. Slower verb learning means that the provision of arguments associated with these verbs could also be limited – though we would require a much more detailed account of the data to be sure of this. In particular we would need to examine the lexical instantiation of arguments occurring with both old and new verbs, in order to determine to what extent the constructions the children are using are item-based. This in turn implies that monthly sampling is likely to be inadequate. For a suitable assay of verb-containing constructions, the longitudinal samples we scrutinise from children with SLI, and from the typically developing children we are comparing them with, will need to be much more dense (Tomasello & Stahl 2004). The speech of these children needs to be sampled at more frequent intervals, and for longer on each occasion. We return to this issue below.

4.3.2 *Aspect markers*

Cantonese grammar has six morphemes which have aspectual meanings (Matthews & Yip 1994: 198). The forms are optional. They are selected by speakers to reflect their perspective on the internal temporal structure of an event, and the absence of an aspect marker does not render a sentence ungrammatical. Two of these forms are perfective, and two imperfective, while the set is completed by a morpheme which denotes repeated or habitual activity (*hoi1*), and another which is described as "delimitative" (*haa5*). When attached to an activity verb this form constrains the time frame of the activity it describes to a very brief period. The two imperfective forms, *gan2* and *zyu6*, are described as "progressive" and "continuous" respectively (Matthews & Yip 1994: 202). (Cantonese morphemes are written in Romanized form. Numerals following the morphemes represent tone values, following the system adopted by the Linguistic Society of Hong Kong, 1994). The *gan2* form applies to dynamic, ongoing activity, while *zyu6* indicates a continuous activity or state. The contrast between the two perfective forms, *zo2* and *gwo3*, hinges on whether the event on which they provide a viewpoint of completion or termination still applies (*zo2*) or has been experienced but does not now hold (*gwo3*).

Studies of aspect in typically developing Cantonese-speaking children are few. Leung (1995) reports on a longitudinal study involving a child who was 21 months old at the outset, and 45 months old when observation ceased. By 21 months this child was using the perfective marker *zo2*, and marking it on nine different verbs. The next aspect markers to appear were the imperfectives *zyu6* (24 months) and *gan2* (39 months). Lee, Wong and Wong (1996) confirm the early appearance of *zo2* and *zyu6*, followed by *gan2*, in two boys followed longitudinally. In both cases *zo2* appeared first, at 21 months for one boy, Bernard and at 23 months for Tsuntsun. For Bernard *zyu6* was observed at 27 months and for Tsuntsun at 25 months. Tsuntsun produced *gan2* at 30 months. The *gwo3* form does not appear in either the Leung or Lee et al. databases. The data are limited, but they do suggest that for Cantonese-speaking children, as for the counterparts learning other languages, the late second and third years of life will see the initial development of grammatical morphemes with

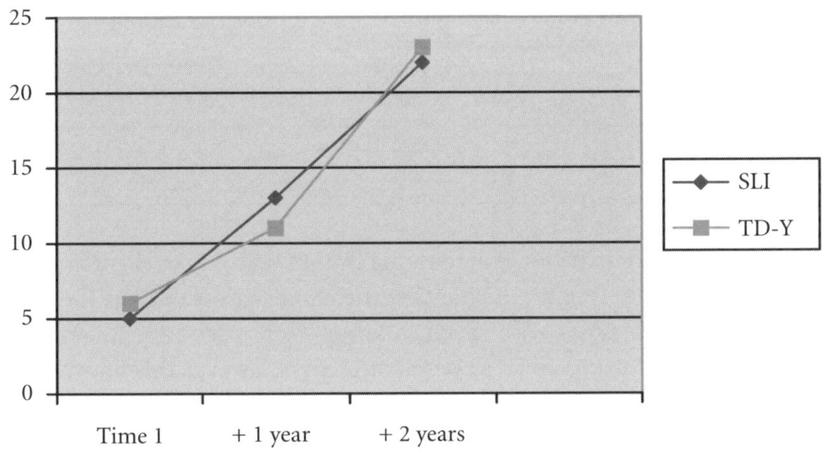

Figure 2. Provision of aspect marker tokens over time in SLI and TD-Y groups

temporal meanings. Cross-sectional studies of the use of aspect markers by Cantonese-speaking children with SLI suggest differences in their control of aspect markers in comparison to typically developing age peers, and younger normal children. Stokes and Fletcher (2000) report differences between SLI and TD-Y groups for one of the perfective markers, *zo2*, while Stokes and Fletcher (2003) found that SLI and age-matched (AM) groups differed on the full range of aspect morphemes. Fletcher, Leonard, Wong and Stokes (in press) compared the performance of an SLI group on *zo2* and *gan2* to that of both TD-Y and AM counterparts, and replicated the earlier results. Here we will turn to the longitudinal database, part of which was used for the 'new verb' analysis, and examine the productivity over time of those aspect markers that appear in the data. The comparison is between SLI and TD-Y groups.

The provision of aspect markers in language samples was explored, in terms both of aspect marker tokens, and in terms of the verbs to which the markers were attached. The data were examined at three time points, separated by a year in each case. Figure 2 shows that the number of aspect tokens supplied by the two groups does not differ across the two year period between the initial and final sample.

However there are differences between the groups in the productivity of the markers. The somewhat conservative criteria for productivity were designed to reduce the influence of item-based utterances. A form was regarded as non-productive if the verb types to which it was attached were equal to verb tokens, and the number of verb tokens was less than 6; and if the verb tokens

Table 1. Productivity over time of aspect markers in SLI and TD-Y groups

	TIME 1		+ ONE YEAR		+ TWO YEARS			
	zo2	*haa5*	*zo2*	*haa5*	*zo2*	*haa5*	*zyu6*	*gwo3*
SLI	N	N	Y	N	Y	Y	N	N
TD-Y	Y	N	Y	N	Y	Y	Y	Y

were less than 6 and distributed across one or two verbs. Like all such criteria, these are arbitrary. It is still possible that the child who produced the perfective form *zo2* seven times with seven different verbs, or seven tokens across two verbs, was still using an item-based strategy. However this approach did identify productivity differences between the groups, as Table 1 shows.

It will be recalled that the average age of the SLI group at the beginning of the sampling is 53 months, and of the TD-Y group, 36 months. Point-by-point comparisons of aspect marker productivity over the two years shows that at no time were the SLI group ahead of the TD-Y group in their command of a specific form. In conformity with the available developmental data, *zo2* is the first form to appear. It is used by both groups at Time 1, but according to our criteria is only productive for the SLI group a year later. And even after two years, one of the imperfective forms (*zyu6*) and the other perfective form (*gwo3*) still remains unproductive for the children in the SLI group.

The salience of aspect forms in Cantonese – they carry a lexical tone and undergo no phonetic reduction – would seem likely to assist their development. The equivalence of the SLI and TD-Y groups in the provision of aspect tokens bears this out. However their optionality, and consequent irregular provision in the input, together with problems in working out the precise function of the different forms, may make it difficult for children with SLI to appreciate the full potential of aspect markers, and so limit their generalizability. Stokes and Fletcher (2000) found evidence for this cross-sectionally. The TD-Y children in that study distributed their *zo2* tokens across 23 verbs; the children with SLI across just 14. And two-thirds of the *zo2* tokens they used were distributed across only three of these 14 verbs: *m4gin2* – "disappear"; *dit3* – "fall"; and *sik6* – "eat". It can be argued that the longitudinal data summarized in Table 2 is similarly suggestive of a more prolonged period of item-by-item learning in children with SLI as compared with younger typically developing children. Of course, as with 'new verbs', the data available, even though it does track performance across time, inhibits full confidence in this conclusion, and for the same reasons. For a complete evaluation of the trajectory from verb islands to abstract constructions, we would require sampling at much more frequent intervals, and more extensive data at each of those intervals. Nevertheless a perspective on typical and atypical development in Cantonese which integrates lexis and syntax appears promising. We now turn to an exploration more generally of the implications of this perspective for assessment and intervention in language impairment.

5. Assessment and intervention from a constructional perspective

5.1 Assessment

We began by observing the significance that research on typical development has had for practice in relation to language impairment. This can be seen in current assessment procedures and in intervention. For example, in an overview of the effectiveness of procedures for grammar facilitation, Fey and Proctor-Williams (2000: 178) enunciate a series of principles concerning successful intervention. The first of these suggests that intervention will be successful to the extent that 'target forms' are more frequent in the input, and the second requires that there is clarification of the semantic correlates of these target forms. These and four remaining principles are directed towards the tense/agreement/auxiliary complex, which is a focus of attention both because it is continually identified as an area of vulnerability for English-speaking children with SLI, and because these areas of the grammar remain part of the computational core of grammars within the Chomskyan tradition. It is clear that the identification of target forms through assessment, and their provision in input in situations where their meanings could be clearly understood, would be mandatory for any successful intervention. However it can be argued that the identification of target forms from a constructional perspective would be fundamentally different – and perhaps a far more difficult prospect – if children do acquire syntax in the way Tomasello (2000a) outlines.

A basic tenet of this alternative approach is that the language children initially acquire is not organized in terms of abstract linguistic categories such as N, VP, or SVO, but is 'almost totally concrete' (Tomasello 2000a: 2). Progress to abstract categories is gradual, relatively unsystematic, and subject presumably to individual variation. Transitivity, as we have already seen, is a case in point. Evidence for the gradual development of an abstract, verb-general transitive construction comes from two directions. Experimental studies involving novel verbs presented in a sentence frame other than transitive (intransitive, imperative) reveal that it is only by about four years of age that the majority of typically developing children demonstrate the ability to generalize the novel verb to a transitive frame (Tomasello 2003:130). And longitudinal studies of speech samples from 12 children between one and three years of age have indicated a selectivity of construction type for particular verbs, and little evidence that children knew how to reliably mark subjects and objects syntactically via pronoun case (Tomasello 2000a:3).

If we extrapolate these findings to pre-schoolers with SLI, it will immediately be apparent that, in evaluating a spontaneous language sample, to label an utterance such as *me draw circle* as SVO is potentially problematic. Even if there were, say, 8 such sentences with different verbs in a sample of 50 utterances, it would still not be legitimate to assume that the child had mastered the transitive construction, for the lexical specificity of the verb argument has to be taken into account. The verb island hypothesis, as an account of the linguistic knowledge of two year olds, claims that they may be working not with abstract syntactic categories, or even participant roles such agent and patient, but such verb-specific elements as (in relation to *draw*), 'drawer' and 'thing drawn'. Accordingly we should be able to identify not only a proliferation of verbs, but a variety of lexical items instantiating the objects of those verbs, in order to assume productivity. These requirements immediately begin to undermine the utility of a language sample of 50 or 100 utterances for the purpose of establishing the current language status of a pre-school child with language impairment. And identifying targets for remediation will be equally problematic. Such a sample can still be used to provide useful summary measures such as MLU or D, but its validity in establishing the point that a child has reached on the path to abstraction of a particular construction is questionable.

From this realization certain conclusions follow. The database for an evaluation of a child's current expressive linguistic status has to be rich. In the (very likely) event that longitudinal data prior to evaluation is not available for the child, an assessment may need to be extended over several data-collection sessions, with analysis of performance paying particular attention to the lexical productivity of constructions of interest. Even so, a definitive judgment on the level of abstraction a child has reached may not be feasible. The evaluation will then need to include elicitation probes designed specifically to assess the generalizability of novel elements. Models for this are available, for transitivity, in e.g. Tomasello and Brooks 1998 (see also Tomasello 2000b). Then, once we extend our gaze from a narrow focus on morphosyntax to constructions that are central to English or Cantonese syntax such as transitives, it becomes clear that what may be a lengthy journey for typically developing children towards abstraction, will be even more arduous for children who are language-impaired. And one-off assessment procedures that apply abstract category labels at the outset, rather than as the outcome of an extended evaluation, may well drastically over-estimate the distance the child with language impairment has traveled. Finally, the target forms to emerge from assessments that are descriptively adequate are likely to be lexically much more specific than we are accustomed to. If for example we find that the child is unable to generalize a causative-inchoative verb (Levin 1993: 27) from its intransitive form (*the ball bounces*) to a transitive version (*he bounced the ball*), target forms might involve a variety of instances of *bounce* and different subjects and direct objects before advancing to other members of this extensive group of alternating verbs in English.

5.2 Intervention

The constructional approach to explaining language development is put forward as a 'usage-based theory'. There are two facets of the role of usage in the theory which are pertinent here. By taking into account the full range of adult language performance, the use of unanalyzable, potentially unanalyzed or partially unanalyzed expressions, which function perfectly well communicatively, is acknowledged. Greetings, idioms, frames such *the more the merrier* (cf. *the fewer the better*) are seen to be as much part of language knowledge as exemplars of more productive constructions. In a unified approach to linguistic expressions, the relevance of this to acquisition is that a child's utterance may appear to be an exemplar of an abstract construction, but instead is for the child at present an unanalyzed expression – though it may well be analyzed later by her, and play a role in the path to abstraction. Usage-based models are also germane to intervention because they use type and token frequency to explain how language development proceeds in the typically developing learner (Tomasello 2003: 107). Token frequency enables the learner to 'entrench' an expression as a whole. So extensive experience of *oh dear*, in the relevant contexts, would allow the 18 month old to store and use the expression appropriately. In the same way a concrete but potentially analyzable expression such as *Where's mummy?* could become entrenched. The usage-based approach then assumes that type frequency is what permits progress towards a construction, where type frequency is defined as 'the number of different forms in which the language learner experiences the expression or some element of the expression' (Tomasello 2003: 107). We may then observe the child progressing from numerous instances of *Where's mummy?* to *Where's grandma?*, *Where's bunny?* etc. The immediate question that arises in relation to the usage-based model is the inability of the child with language impairment, by definition, to take advantage of the information available in input.

This is of course not a problem only for an approach to language impairment from a constructional direction. Intervention, however it is informed theoretically, and however confident in its choice of intervention targets, still has to find a way to implement its goals. And it has to achieve these goals in the face of a language learning mechanism that has already demonstrated its reluctance to take full advantage of the ambient language environment. There is an extensive literature on procedures for facilitating intervention goals (see Fey & Proctor-Williams 2000 and references therein). The procedures – didactic teaching exercises, recasting, modeling, elicited imitation – are theory-neutral. Fey and Proctor-Williams conclude that 'there is no one procedure [that] will optimize the development of difficult morphological and syntactic forms among children with SLI' (2000: 191).

This assertion may well reflect the state of the art, but the two aspects of the usage-based model we have outlined hold out hope for a more informed approach to the role of input in typically developing children, and from there to the deficiencies in children with language impairment, and perhaps more effective approaches to remediation. Within dense longitudinal databases it should possible to quantify the role of input tokens in the establishment of specific expressions, and of input types in the development of constructions. Work along these lines is already under way. Rowland, Pine, Lieven and Theakston (2003), in an analysis of the language to and from 12 two to three year olds, found that the acquisition order of wh-questions was predictable from the frequency with which particular wh-words and verbs occurred in the children's input. (See also Wong et al. 2004 for evidence on the role of input frequency in interrogative performance in Cantonese-speaking children with SLI.) The more we know about input benchmarks necessary to entrench expressions and constructions in typically developing children, the more informed our intervention procedures can become. These benchmarks will include, in addition to frequency, information on lexical variation in target expressions and the nature of the contexts in which input expressions occur.

6. Conclusion

The constructional approach has the merit first of all of forcing us to a reappraisal of typical language development. The emphasis on item-based expressions, the extended route to constructional competence, and the functional role of input provides a robust counter to a view of language development as the unfolding of a genetically determined blueprint, with input as a necessary condition for success but of limited influence on the course of events. The constructional approach reminds us that successful language development, while achievable in any language by the vast majority of infants, is nevertheless a complex and lengthy process. This in turn helps us to keep language impairment in perspective, as an even more laborious process which may not ultimately be completely successful. And if we see impairment as the consequence of a less than optimum interaction between an organism and the ambient language environment, we can ask what it is about the organism or the environment that inhibits development. As we have indicated, further work on the role of input frequency may play a part in answering this question.

The focus on the transition from item-based expressions to constructions, sometimes across a period of years, also requires us to examine the role of lexis in the evolution of a mature grammar and then in our assessment procedures, and the intervention targets that these identify. We have already reviewed studies of limited lexical diversity in Cantonese-speaking children with SLI, both generally and in relation to verbs. There is extensive research on lexical deficiencies in English-speaking children with language impairment (see Leonard & Deevy 2004 for a summary). As with the Cantonese-speaking children, at least some of these lexical deficits could cause what Leonard and Deevy refer to as 'collateral damage' to the establishment of constructions, since all lexical items appear in some syntactic context.

Finally, the methods that construction grammar entails, for a proper exploration of its predictions – dense, longitudinally organized language samples, and experimental probes for constructional generalization – should influence new approaches to both research and assessment for children with SLI. It is clear that we need to know a great deal more than we do about the progress of language learning in these children over time. We also require assessment procedures which give us a better chance of identifying where the children stand in the developmental course, and of devising intervention accordingly.

Language development in Down syndrome and fragile X syndrome

Current research and implications for theory and practice*

Leonard Abbeduto and Robin S. Chapman

In this chapter, we review research on the development of language in Down syndrome and fragile X syndrome, which are the two most common (known) genetic causes of mental retardation (Dykens, Hodapp, & Finucane 2000). In doing so, we address three goals. First, we hope to provide a concise but comprehensive characterization of the profile of language development associated with each syndrome. More extended reviews of the literatures on these syndromes can be found in Chapman (2003) and Murphy and Abbeduto (2003). Second, we argue that the data on language development in these two syndromes are relevant to long-standing controversies in the study of language development more generally. These controversies are embodied in the contrasting claims of the modularity and interactionist accounts of development (Abbeduto, Evans, & Dolan 2001a; Chapman 2000). The modularity account presumes strong innate constraints on development, a rather minimal and circumscribed role for experience, and a relative independence of language development from other facets of development. In contrast, the social-interactionist account supposes intimate bidirectional influences between language development and nonlinguistic developments in other domains (e.g., social cognition) and a critical role for experiences, particularly experiences in social interaction with caregivers and other supportive, competent language users. Third, we briefly sketch some of the implications for clinical practice of the empirical research we consider.

The chapter is organized as follows. First, we consider research on Down syndrome and its implications for developmental theory and clinical practice.

Next, we consider research on fragile X syndrome and its implications. We conclude by briefly considering the value of integrating research on the two syndromes.

1. Language development and the behavioral phenotype of Down syndrome

Down syndrome results from a third copy of all or part of chromosome 21, with its attendant consequences of gene dosage effects on fetal development, physiology, and brain functioning. Extra copies of the 225 genes (Hattori, Fujiyama, Taylor, Watanabe, Yada, Park, Toyoda, Ishii, Totoki, Choi, Groner, Soeda, Ohki, Takagi, Sakaki, Taudien, Blechschmidt, Polley, Menzel, Delabar, Kumpf, Lehmann, Patterson, Reichwald, Rump, Schillhabel, Schudy, Zimmermann, Rosenthal, Kudoh, Schibuya, Kawasaki, Asakawa, Shintani, Sasaki, Nagamine, Mitsuyama, Antonarakis, Minoshima, Shimizu, Nordsiek, Hornischer, Brant, Scharfe, Schon, Desario, Reichelt, Kauer, Blocker, Ramser, Beck, Klages, Hennig, Riesselmann, Dagand, Haaf, Wehrmeyer, Borzym, Gardiner, Nizetic, Francis, Lehrach, Reinhardt, Yaspo; Chromosome 21 mapping and sequencing consortium 2000)[1] on chromosome 21 have more than 80 known physical and behavioral consequences (Epstein, Korenberg, Anneren, Antonarakis, Ayme, Courchesne, Epstein, Fowler, Groner, Huret, Kempter, Lott, Lubin, Magenis, Opitz, Patterson, Priest, Pueschel, Rapoport, Sinet, Tanzi, & de la Cruz 1991; Korenberg, Chen, Schipper, Sun, Gonsky, Gerwehr, Carpenter, Daumer, Dignan, Disteche Graham Jr., Hugdins, McGillivray, Miyazaki, Ogasawara, Park, Pagon, Pueschel, Sack, Say, Schuffenhauer, Soukup, & Yamanaka 1991; Reeves, Baxter, & Richtsmeier 2001). Thus, Down syndrome differs from a single-gene alteration, as in fragile X syndrome, or a small set of affected genes, as in Williams syndrome, in the number of potential genetic correlates for behavioral consequences. Phenotypic characteristics in the population thus reflect the over-expression of multiple genes on chromosome 21, the interaction of differing alleles with one another, and the genetic makeup of other chromosome pairs.

Intensive research on language and cognitive development in children and adolescents with Down syndrome has given us a detailed picture of the behavioral phenotype associated with the syndrome, its developmental emergence, and the wide individual variation in development that can occur (Abbeduto, Pavetto, Kesin, Weissman, Karadottir, O'Brien, & Cawthon 2001b; Chapman & Hesketh 2000; Miller 1999; Roizen 2001). This research has also revealed a number of factors that affect language learning in specific domains (Chapman 2003; Chapman, Hesketh, & Kistler 2002).

2. The emerging behavioral phenotype in Down syndrome

Infancy (0–4 years). Nonverbal cognitive delays on both standardized and Piagetian tasks emerge at ages 0 to 2 years and accelerate at ages 3 and 4; social skills appear commensurate with mental age, as does comprehension of vocabulary (Dykens, Hodapp, & Evans 1994). Studies of young children with Down syndrome make clear that problems emerge in prelinguistic communication, with less frequent nonverbal requesting behavior than children of comparable mental age (Mundy, Kasari, Sigman, & Ruskin 1995), and continue with the slower accumulation of productive vocabulary relative to mental age, even when signing is taken into account (Miller 1995). The proportion of preschool children with Down syndrome showing significant delays in productive vocabulary development increases with age (Miller 1999). Expressive language also lags behind social skills (Dykens, Hodapp, & Evans 1994). Comparison to typically developing children matched on overall language age shows no difference in use of gestures but fewer two-word combinations on the part of children with Down syndrome (Iverson, Longobardi, & Caselli 2003). Speech, too, is affected in Down syndrome, with a slower transition from babbling to speech and poorer intelligibility (Stoel-Gammon 1997).

Childhood (4–12 years). Expressive language delays in vocabulary, utterance length, utterance complexity, and grammatical morphology continue in childhood relative to receptive vocabulary, syntax comprehension, and nonverbal cognition (Chapman & Hesketh 2000; Cunningham, Glenn, Wilkinson, & Sloper 1985). Speech development shows a longer period of phonological errors and more variability in production (Stoel-Gammon 1997). Intelligibility of the speech produced by children with Down syndrome is a frequent concern of parents (Kumin 1994). Nonverbal cognitive development reveals specific deficits in verbal working memory (Marcell & Weeks 1988). Socially, children with Down syndrome have more behavior problems than siblings without Down syndrome, but fewer compared to other children with other types of cognitive disability (Stores, Stores, Fellows, & Buckley 1998). Problems that do occur tend to be anxiety, depression, and withdrawal, and these increase with age (Dykens & Kasari 1997).

Examination of social skills shows some specific deficits despite the reported high levels of sociability displayed by children with Down syndrome on average: skill in emotion recognition is delayed (Kasari, Freeman, & Hughes 2001), especially for fear and surprise (Wishart & Pitcairn 2000); and preference for social interaction rather than object manipulation is more prolonged developmentally than one would expect on the basis of other cognitive tasks (Kasari, Sigman, Mundy, & Yirmiya 1990; Kasari, Freeman, Mundy, & Sigman 1995). There is also evidence of excessive delays in some facets of understanding the mental states of other people (Abbeduto et al. 2001b; Yirmiya, Erel, Shaked, & Solomonica-Levi 1998; Zelazo, Burack, Benedetto, & Frye 1996). Children with Down syndrome respond more often to distress in others by looking to them more, and offering more comfort, than typically developing children matched for mental age; but are less likely to feel the same emotion as the protagonist in hypothetical situations (Kasari, Freeman, & Bass 2003).

Adolescence (*12–18 years*). Comprehension of words appears more advanced than comprehension of syntax and nonverbal mental age, when measures of vocabulary such as the Peabody Picture Vocabulary Test are used (Chapman, Schwartz, & Kay-Raining Bird 1991). More recent research (Chapman 2003), however, shows that the advantage relative to mental age disappears when a vocabulary test selected for conceptual difficulty, rather than frequency of occurrence (e.g. the vocabulary subtest of the Test of Auditory Comprehension of Language-3), is used, although grammatical morpheme and elaborated sentence comprehension are poorer yet (Abbeduto, Murphy, Cawthon, Richmond, Weissman, Karadottir, & O'Brien 2003; Chapman et al. 1991). Comprehension of syntax lags nonverbal cognition in adolescence (Rosin, Swift, Bless, & Vetter 1988). Longitudinal study shows actual loss of skills in receptive syntax in some individuals through late adolescence and the beginning of young adulthood (Chapman et al. 2002).

Expressive language deficits relative to nonverbal mental age persist, with grammatical morpheme production more deficient than predicted on the basis of MLU or the lexicon (Vicari, Caselli, & Tonucci 2000). Grammatical and lexical verb use per utterance is less frequent than would expect based on MLU, but lexical diversity of narrative samples is greater (Hesketh & Chapman 1998). The proportion of verbs that are metalinguistic or metacognitive, however, is significantly less than MLU controls (Hesketh & Chapman 1998), a finding which may be related to earlier emerging problems in emotion recognition or to differences in parent input (Tingley, Gleason, & Hooshyar 1994).

Importantly, however, adolescents continue to make progress, albeit it slow, in utterance length and sentence complexity (Chapman, Seung, Schwartz, & Kay-Raining Bird 1998; Chapman et al. 2002). Longer utterances as measured by MLU are associated with more complex sentence structures, and complex sentence use is as advanced as MLU-matched controls (Thordardottir, Chapman, & Wagner 2002; Grela 2003). Speech intelligibility continues to be a concern, with more variability in fundamental frequency, rate control, and placement of sentential stress than expected. Problems of auditory verbal short-term memory persist (Seung & Chapman 2000), and visual short-term memory begins to lag visual cognition on tests of these skills (Chapman et al. 1991). Social development continues, with fewer behavioral problems than peers with other cognitive disabilities (Pueschel 1996).

Young adulthood. Skill patterns in young adulthood (19–27 years) are similar to those of late adolescence. Longitudinal study shows loss of syntax comprehension skill (Chapman et al. 2002). Progress in expressive language learning continues and includes the acquisition of complex syntax (Thordardottir et al. 2002). Speech problems, still frequent, include a higher incidence of hypernasality and stuttering (Kumin 1994), but intelligibility improves with chronological age and hearing status (Chapman et al. 1998). Behavioral symptoms of dementia are not evident in young adulthood; indeed, they only begin to emerge at age 50 for approximately half the individuals studied, linked to the increase in beta-amyloid protein associated with three copies of the APP gene on chromosome 21 (Silverman & Wisniewski 1999) and the moderating influence of APOE alleles.

3. Predictors of individual difference

Although Down syndrome is associated with a typical behavioral phenotype, it is important to acknowledge that the syndrome is accompanied by wide individual differences in developmental rate. What predicts the individual variations? Evidence from language learning in children with Down syndrome can partially illuminate a long-standing controversy in theories of language acquisition: the question of whether nonverbal cognition determines language learning rate. The argument that nonverbal cognition should predict a significant proportion of the variance in language learning stems from the interactionist theory's belief that general cognitive mechanisms drive language learning, rather than language-specific ones (Abbeduto et al. 2001a). However, amount of language input, enriched learning environments, social skills, motor skills, working memory skills, and hearing status, among other variables, will also contribute to language learning, in the interactionist account (Chapman 2000). A modular view, in contrast, predicts a reduced correlation of nonverbal cognition and language measures, and synchrony among the language measures.

Predictors of individual difference in comprehension skills (both syntactic and lexical) include chronological age and nonverbal cognition; hearing contributes significant explained variance to the measure of grammatical morphology comprehension (Chapman et al. 1991). Longitudinal evaluation, with the addition of auditory working memory to the predictor set, and separation of nonverbal cognition into pattern analysis and visual short-term memory skills, reveals that the visual and auditory working memory, together with chronological age, are the best predictors of overall syntax comprehension; and the rate of change in visual working memory skill predicts rate of change in syntax comprehension (Chapman et al. 2002). Auditory short-term memory skills do not change over this period, an observation also reported by Laws and Gunn (2004). Thus, cognitive variables predict language learning, as the interactionist view would expect; but they are the variables of working memory, rather than visual pattern analysis skill.

The best model for predicting individual difference in longitudinal measures of expressive language skill, as indexed by MLU, contains syntax comprehension at study start, to predict production at study start; and slope of comprehension change, to predict rate of expressive language growth. How can it be that losses in syntax comprehension and gains in syntax expression simultaneously occur? One possibility is that language input, to the extent that it is responsive to what individuals say rather than what they understand, will be targeted at the lower production level and hence prove less useful to continued development of syntax comprehension skills. A second possibility is that the shift to vocational training in mid-adolescence, and the end of language intervention in educational programs, reduces the overall effectiveness of the language learning environment, but that expressive syntax growth can continue, for a time, to take advantage of the greater syntactic knowledge in comprehension. In either case, we need to examine the language learning environment for older adolescents and young adults with Down syndrome.

4. Implications for modular vs. interactive theories of language acquisition

How does language learning come apart? The study of specific behavioral phenotypes also assists in assessing the relative merits of modular vs. interactionist theories of language acquisition, which imply different patterns of strength and deficit (see, e.g., Chapman 2000). In particular, modular theories would imply that a particular linguistic domain could reflect a relative strength or weakness, and syntax has been proposed as the locus of the deficit in Down syndrome (Epstein et al. 1991). This view would imply deficits in both comprehension and production in the affected domain across the developmental span. Interactionist theories, in contrast, link linguistic strengths and deficits to language learning in social, emotional, and cognitive domains, working memory systems, comprehension and production requirements, and the communicative contexts encountered (e.g. Chapman et al. 1992; Elman, Bates, Johnson, Karmiloff-Smith, Parisi, & Plunkett 1996; MacWhinney 1999). The interactionist view would thus predict that deficits in nonverbal domains, short-term memory, or long-term store would have developmentally changing effects on phenotypic profiles.

The evidence just reviewed on language development in individuals with Down syndrome supports an interactionist rather than a modular perspective (Chapman & Hesketh 2000). Syntax is indeed identified as an area of deficit in children, but particularly in production, rather than comprehension, until late adolescence, when losses in syntax comprehension are encountered. Mean length of utterance is shorter in individuals with Down syndrome than one would expect on the basis of their nonverbal cognitive skills, and the grammatical constructions observed at each utterance length are typical of those found in MLU, rather than mental age, comparison groups (Thordardottir et al. 2002). The content of stories narrated after watching short wordless videos (Boudreau & Chapman 2000) or wordless picture books (Miles & Chapman 2002), however, is greater than that in the MLU-matched group, and similar to that of the group matched for syntax comprehension skill.

Grammatical morphology in production shows the most severe deficit, including more errors and omissions than the MLU-matched group (Chapman et al. 1998; Eadie, Fey, Douglas, & Parsons 2002). The deficit extends beyond tense inflections to include non-tense grammatical morphemes (Eadie et al. 2002). Comprehension of grammatical morphology, however, is consistent with nonverbal cognitive level unless hearing impairment limits comprehension (Chapman et al. 2002). Finally, the developmental trajectory for intelligibility improves with age and hearing status (Chapman, Seung, Schwartz, & Kay-Raining Bird 2000).

Thus, the trajectories for growth of syntax comprehension and production separate, and within language production, the trajectory of thematic and plot content separates from sentence form, with grammatical morphology lagging even further behind. In other words, language learning in Down syndrome fractionates along the lines of comprehension vs. production, content vs. form, and grammatical elements vs. grammatical structure.

5. The critical period hypothesis

The Critical Period Hypothesis of language learning is another major theoretical claim that can be evaluated in individual with cognitive disabilities. The question is whether there is a limit to the developmental period in which language can be easily learned; the onset of adolescence has been thought to be the end of the period. In her work with younger adolescents with Down syndrome, Fowler (Fowler, Gelman, & Gleitman 1994) reported plateauing of expressive language, a finding consistent with a belief in a critical period. Longitudinal research by Chapman and colleagues, however, has documented continued progress in expressive language learning throughout adolescence and young adulthood (Chapman et al. 2002). The difference in the two findings appears to be due to the method of language sampling: Fowler used a conversational, rather than narrative, sample; the latter offers more opportunity for later-learned syntactic structures to be used. Additionally, the Chapman et al. work included a larger, and older, sample of adolescents as well as young adults.

The finding of continued progress in expressive syntax in adolescence has implications for our understanding of the nature of "critical periods" observed in typical second language learners. If maturation is not a factor, as the data from the group with Down syndrome suggest, then perhaps it is the amount of first language learning itself (or learning in other domains that overtakes the usual neural locus of language) that ultimately makes learning a second language more difficult, rather than the age of the learner.

6. Implications for clinical practice

We have reviewed evidence for a specific behavioral phenotype in language and cognition for individuals with Down syndrome that includes deficits in expressive language syntax, especially grammatical morphology, and deficits in phonological working memory; as well as strengths in lexical comprehension. We find that both auditory and visual short-term memory measures, and chronological age, predict individual differences in syntax comprehension; syntax comprehension, in turn, predicts the course of syntax production.

There is no evidence of a critical period in adolescence; rather, losses in syntax comprehension, and gains in expressive syntax. Hearing status predicts intelligibility and grammatical morpheme comprehension. Visual support for story construction differentially increases expressive syntax for individuals with Down syndrome.

From this evidence, several implications for clinical practice can be drawn. First, goals in comprehension and production should have in mind the individual's differing developmental levels in the two domains. If all intervention work is addressed to production levels, future progress may be compromised. Second, hearing status, even within the range of mild loss, plays a critical role in intelligibility and grammatical morpheme comprehension; hearing should be monitored and aided, if needed. Third, language intervention work should continue in adolescence and young adulthood, focused on both production and comprehension, for these individuals are still developing language skill. The use of visual support for storytelling may be particularly helpful in supporting more complex syntax production. Additionally, a life-long learning approach to language and literacy skills is warranted.

7. Language development and the behavioral phenotype of fragile X syndrome

Fragile X syndrome is the leading inherited cause of mental retardation and is second only to Down syndrome as a genetic cause of mental retardation (Hagerman 1999). Fragile X syndrome is caused by a mutation in a single gene (FMR1) located on the X chromosome (Brown 2002). In the full mutation, a repetitive sequence of trinucleotides (i.e., the CGG repeats), which is typically characterized by 54 or fewer repeats, expands to more than 200 (Oostra 1996). This expansion results in a silencing of the gene, which blocks production of its associated protein (Oostra & Willemsen 2003). This protein (FMRP) has been found to play a critical role in experience-dependent maturation and functioning of neural synapses (Greenough, Klintsova, Irwin, Galvez, Bates, & Weiler 2001). In contrast to Down syndrome, then, the problem in fragile X syndrome is one of gene under-expression rather than over-expression. Also in contrast to Down syndrome, in which the genetic anomaly has the same consequences for affected males and females, fragile X syndrome differentially affects the sexes. Thus, the prevalence of affected individuals is 1 in 4,000 births in males and 1 in 8,000 in females (Crawford, Acuna, & Sherman 2001). Moreover, whereas males with the full mutation typically meet diagnostic criteria for mental retardation, only half of females with the full mutation do so, with the remainder having normal-range IQs, but learning disabilities or social affective involvement (Mazzocco 2000).

The behavioral phenotype of fragile X syndrome has been intensely investigated for the past three or more decades, although research on language has been sparse compared to that on Down syndrome (Murphy & Abbeduto 2003). Nevertheless, there are features of the fragile X syndrome phenotype that distinguish it from Down syndrome in ways that are likely to have consequences for language development (Murphy & Abbeduto 2003). Most notable in this regard are the substantially higher rates of psychopathology observed in fragile X syndrome compared to Down syndrome (Mazzocco 2000). The behaviors associated with these psychopathologies, which are described further below, can lead the individual with fragile X syndrome to avoid or have difficulties with participation in social interaction and thereby interfere with the acquisition and use of language (Cornish, Sudhalter, & Turk 2004; Murphy & Abbeduto 2005). In contrast, individuals with Down syndrome are highly sociable and keenly interested in social interaction (Kasari et al. 1990, 1995), although they may lack some important social skills that their mental age-matched typical peers possess (Abbeduto et al. 2001; Kasari et al. 2003; Yirmiya, Erel, Shaked, & Solomonica-Levi 1998; Zelazo, Burack, Benedetto, & Frye 1996). This difference in psychopathology, particularly in the social-affective realm, suggests that comparisons between fragile X syndrome and Down syndrome may be informative about theoretical controversies concerning the mechanisms of language development, especially those regarding the role of social experience (Murphy & Abbeduto 2005). In this section, we briefly describe what is known about the behavioral phenotype and development of language in fragile X syndrome. In doing so, we have distinguished between research on males and females only to the extent that that there are different findings for the two (i.e., rather than simply differences in the degree of affectedness).

8. The emerging behavioral phenotype in fragile X syndrome

In contrast to the case for Down syndrome, developmental changes in the behavioral phenotype associated with fragile X syndrome have not been well characterized (Murphy & Abbeduto 2005). In part, this reflects the fact that the diagnosis of fragile X syndrome is not confirmed until near the age of three or four years on average (Bailey, Skinner, Hatton, & Roberts 2000a) despite the fact that many of these children exhibit delays during the first year of life (Mirrett, Bailey, Roberts, & Hatton 2004). As a result of this delay in diagnosis, studies of behavioral development in infancy are rare and thus, a critical portion of the life span is unexplored for this population. It is also the case, however, that many studies of the behavioral phenotype of fragile X syndrome, especially those focused on language, have involved samples of affected individuals that are heterogeneous with respect to age, with comparisons made to various control samples but with little attention to age-related differences within the samples (Murphy & Abbeduto 2003, in press). This lack of a developmental perspective is particularly problematic in light of the fact that the physical stigmata associated with syndrome, including the elongated face, prominent ears, and (among boys) enlarged testicles, are actually exacerbated with age (Hagerman 1999). Moreover, there is now convincing evidence that the rate of cognitive development, at least as reflected in IQ, slows during late childhood and adolescence in both males and females with fragile X syndrome (Dykens, Hodapp, Ort, Finucane, Shapiro, & Leckman 1989a; Hagerman, Schreiner, Kemper, Wittenberger, Zahn, & Habicht 1989). More studies charting the longitudinal trajectory of language in fragile X syndrome are required before we can fully understand the mechanisms of development in this population.

Development in childhood. Studies employing gross measures of language that summarize performance across the many domains of language (e.g., vocabulary, syntax) have generally found that delays in language during childhood are no more severe than observed in other domains, such as nonverbal cognition, at least for individuals with fragile X syndrome who do not also meet diagnostic criteria for autism (Bailey, Hatton, Mesibov, & Ament 2000b). Such summary measures, however, may obscure the existence of varying degrees of delay and differing trajectories across the different components of language (Abbeduto & Murphy 2004). Indeed, the need for attempting a more nuanced characterization of language is supported by the findings of a longitudinal investigation conducted by Roberts, Mirrett and Burchinal (2001). These investigators found that between the ages of two and seven years, males with fragile X syndrome displayed greater delays relative to their typical age-matched peers in expressive language than in receptive language. In particular, the rate of development was one-third the typical rate in language expression and one-half the rate in the domain of receptive language for the boys with fragile X syndrome. This advantage of reception over expression, however, appears to diminish, at least for some individuals with fragile X syndrome, in adolescence and adulthood (Abbeduto et al. 2000; Madison, George, & Moeschler 1986).

The profile of delays is even less clear for other linguistic distinctions (Abbeduto & Hagerman 1997). In a study of three, 10- to 14-year-old males with fragile X syndrome, Paul, Cohen, Breg, Watson and Herman (1984) documented delays in the syntactic maturity of the boys' conversational language that exceeded their delays in nonverbal cognition. In a study of a single family affected by fragile X syndrome, Madison et al. (1986) found that the only young girl in their sample similarly achieved an MLU in conversation that was substantially below expectations based on her cognitive or receptive language ability. In contrast, Ferrier, Bashir, Meryash, Johnston and Wolff (1991) found no differences between the conversational syntax of males with fragile X syndrome and typically developing males matched to them on age and cognitive level; however, the groups included both children and adults, with no analyses conducted to examine possible age differences.

In summary, results to date suggest that children with fragile X syndrome have especially severe deficits in expressive language. At least some children with fragile X syndrome have especially severe delays in syntax, although it is not clear whether the majority of children with fragile X syndrome display such asynchrony between syntax and cognition. Finally, there have been no studies focused on other important domains of language (e.g., lexical ability, pragmatics) in children with fragile X syndrome (Abbeduto & Hagerman 1997).

Development in adolescence and adulthood. There is evidence from several longitudinal investigations that language in fragile X syndrome, like cognition, is characterized by a declining rate of development, or increasing delay, in later childhood and early adolescence for both males (Bailey et al. 1998; Dykens, Hodapp, Ort, & Leckman 1993; Fisch, Holden, Carpenter, Howard-Peebles, Maddalena, Pandya, & Nance 1999; Freund, Peebles, Aylward, & Reiss 1995; Prouty, Rogers, Stevenson, Dean, Palmer, Simensen, Coston, & Schwartz 1988; Roberts et al. 2001) and females (Dyer-Friedman, Glaser, Hessel, Johnston, Taylor, Wisbeck, & Reiss 2002). In these studies, however, the measures of language have been quite broad (e.g., verbal IQ) thereby making it impossible to determine whether the trajectory of development is variable across different domains, with some domains showing more pronounced declines in rate of growth than other domains (Murphy & Abbeduto 2003).

Cross-sectional comparisons with typically developing individuals and other clinical groups matched on various dimensions of behavioral development (e.g., nonverbal mental age) suggest that, in contrast to the findings for childhood, developments in many domains of language keep pace with nonlinguistic cognitive achievements during adolescence and adulthood. Lexical development has been found to be synchronous with cognitive ability in males and females with fragile X syndrome (Abbeduto et al. 2003; Paul, Dykens, Leckman, Watson, Breg, & Cohen 1987), although the emphasis in studies to date has been largely on the learning of concrete vocabulary and on current knowledge rather than on the nature of the strategies used to learn the meanings of new words (Abbeduto & Hagerman 1997).

Syntactic development, whether measured receptively (Abbeduto et al. 2003) or expressively (Abbeduto et al. 2000; Paul et al. 1987), is synchronous with nonverbal cognitive development in fragile X syndrome on average. Nevertheless, there do appear to be important individual differences in this regard. This is suggested by case studies of a few affected individuals who were found to make more rapid progress in syntax than in nonverbal cognition (Madison et al. 1986).

Together, the findings on lexical and syntactic development suggest that adolescents and young adults with fragile X syndrome acquire the linguistic tools needed to be successful communicators at a rate consistent with their rate of (nonlinguistic) cognitive growth. There also is evidence that the perceptual and oral-motor capabilities needed to hear and produce speech, although impaired relative to chronological age expectations, have developed to a mental age-appropriate level by adolescence (Abbeduto 2004).

In contrast to the results of studies focused on linguistic "tools," studies of various dimensions of language use in social interaction paint a picture of especially severe delay during adolescence and adulthood. Thus, perseveration (i.e., self-repetition of words, phrases, and topics) and the production of tangential language (i.e., utterances that are only loosely related in content to the conversational topic) have been found to be especially frequent in the language of adolescents and adults with fragile X syndrome (Abbeduto & Hagerman 1997; Mirrett, Roberts, & Price 2003; Murphy & Abbeduto 2003). Indeed, the rate of perseverative and tangential language distinguishes males with fragile X syndrome not only from typically developing age peers, but also from age- and developmental level-matched peers with other developmental disabilities, including autism (Belser & Sudhalter 1995, 2001; Sudhalter, Cohen, Silverman, & Wolf-Schein 1990; Sudhalter, Scarborough, & Cohen 1991; Wolf-Schein, Cohen, Fisch, Brown, & Jenkins 1987). Although several methodological limitations of the studies in this area complicate interpretation (Murphy & Abbeduto 2003, 2005), the findings are consistent in documenting an especially severe problem in these domains.

Adolescence and adults with fragile X syndrome also have special difficulty producing utterances in a way that makes their intended referents clear to their listeners. In particular, Abbeduto and his colleagues (Abbeduto & Murphy 2004) found that when describing novel referents to another person, adolescents and young adults with fragile X syndrome often used the same description for different referents, and they did so significantly more often than typically developing 3- to 8-year-olds matched to them on nonverbal mental age. The youth with fragile X syndrome also were more likely than the typically developing comparison children to change their description of the referents, even when those descriptions were successful, as they recurred during the interaction. The failure to create one-to-one mappings of descriptions and referents and to retain successful descriptions will result in discourse that is difficult for others to understand (Abbeduto & Murphy 2004).

Not just the speaker role, but also the listener role, poses especially serious challenges for adolescents and adults with fragile X syndrome. In particular, they are less likely to recognize and take corrective action when they fail to understand a message addressed to them than are mental age-matched typically developing peers (Abbeduto & Murphy 2004). This is true even when the comprehension problem results from the inclusion in the message of an unfamiliar word, an ambiguous noun phrase, or a noun phrase that has no identifiable referent. Such failures are likely to "snowball" during an interaction, making comprehension and participation increasingly difficult as the interaction proceeds (Abbeduto & Murphy 2004).

In summary, although adolescents and adults with fragile X syndrome have many of the linguistic tools they need to participate at reasonably high (i.e., mental age-appropriate levels) in linguistic interactions, they often fail to do so; instead, they perseverate, produce tangential utterances, produce messages whose referents are difficult to determine, and they fail to resolve comprehension problems when in the role of listener. In the next sections, we consider some of the factors that might account for this profile of language development.

9. Predictors of individual difference

The behavioral phenotype of fragile X syndrome includes cognitive limitations and various behaviors reflective of psychopathology. Although mental retardation is characteristic of virtually all males and many females with the full FMR1 mutation, some cognitive skills are more impaired than are others (Mirrett et al. 2003). Areas of special challenge include the processing of sequential information (Burack, Shulman, Katzir, Schaap, Brennan, Iarocci, Wilansky, & Amir 1999; Dykens, Hodapp, & Leckman 1989), arithmetic (Freund & Reiss 1991), and short-term memory (Freund & Reiss 1991). Areas of relative cognitive strength include the processing of simultaneous information (Dykens et al. 1987) and long-term memory, especially for holistic spatial information (Freund & Reiss 1991).

As noted previously, fragile X syndrome is also characterized by high rates of psychopathology. The psychopathology includes hyperarousal (Wisbeck, Huffman, Freund, Gunnar, Davis, & Reiss 2000), hyperactivity and attentional problems (Baumgardner, Reiss, Freund, & Abrams 1995; Bregman, Leckman, & Ort 1988; Dykens et al. 1989; Freund, Reiss, & Abrahms 1993; Mazzocco, Pennington, & Hagerman 1993), social anxiety (Bregman et al. 1988), and gaze avoidance (Cohen, Vietze, Sudhalter, Jenkins, & Brown 1989). Autistic-like behaviors are also frequent in fragile X syndrome (Feinstein & Reiss 2001); indeed, between 10% and 40% of affected individuals have a co-morbid diagnosis of autism (Demark, Feldman, & Holden 2003). The behaviors and limitations associated with these forms of psychopathology are likely to interfere with language learning and use within the contexts of social interaction (Belser & Sudhalter 1995; Cohen 1995; Cornish et al. 2004; Murphy & Abbeduto 2003, 2005).

Few longitudinal studies have been conducted to examine the predictive relationships between various aspects of the behavioral phenotype of fragile X syndrome and the subsequent development of language. In one of the few studies to do so (Roberts et al. 2001), it was found that cognitive ability (as reflected in IQ) predicted rate of growth in both expressive and receptive language for young boys with fragile X syndrome. This is consistent with research on mental retardation more generally: general cognitive ability appears to constrain many aspects of language development (Rosenberg & Abbeduto 1993).

In contrast to the scarcity of longitudinal studies, there have been several cross-sectional studies that have uncovered concurrent relationships between various aspects of the behavioral phenotype of fragile X syndrome and language development. Thus, perseverative and tangential language is correlated with level of physiological arousal, at least in males (Belser & Sudhalter 1995); effectiveness in talking about referents is negatively correlated with the severity of attentional problems (Abbeduto & Murphy 2004); and the ability to resolve comprehension problems is correlated with achievements in social cognition (Abbeduto & Murphy 2004). Although such correlations are consistent with the notion that language learning and use are shaped by psychopathology at least in part through the latter's impact on social interaction, longitudinal tests of these relationships are needed to unambiguously determine the direction of causation (Murphy & Abbeduto 2005).

There is also emerging evidence that the course of language development is very different in individuals with fragile X syndrome who do and do not have a co-morbid diagnosis of autism. In particular, Philofsky, Hepburn, Hayes, Hagerman and Rogers (2004) have found that children with both diagnoses have more substantial deficits in receptive language than do children who have only a diagnosis of fragile X syndrome. Similar findings have been obtained by Murphy, Abbeduto, Giles, Bruno, Richmond and Schroeder (2004). In addition, Bailey et al. (2000b) found that the profile of impairments in children with both a fragile X syndrome and autism diagnosis is similar to that observed in children with only autism (e.g., communication is more impaired than are many other domains of behavioral functioning). At the same time, Bailey et al. (2000b) found that children with fragile X syndrome who did not meet diagnostic criteria for autism displayed more synchrony in their development across the behavioral domains examined.

In summary, various aspects of language learning and use are predicted by cognitive ability, social-cognitive ability, and various forms of psychopathology and maladaptive behavior. Many of these relationships, however, are concurrent, leaving questions about the direction of causation unanswered.

10. Implications for modular vs. interactive theories of language acquisition

Three sets of findings in the literature on fragile X syndrome argue against a modular account of language and in favor of accounts that ascribe an important role to more general learning mechanisms and experience, especially experience within the context of social interaction, such as emergentism (Abbeduto et al. 2001). First, are the findings reviewed in the previous section describing both longitudinal and concurrent relationships between language and various measures of nonlinguistic dimensions of the behavioral phenotype, such as cognitive ability, social-cognitive ability, and psychopathology. Such relationships suggest that either there is a common causal mechanism for the linguistic and nonlinguistic domains examined or achievements in one domain are necessary for, or facilitative of, achievements in the others. Thus, these relationships are at odds with the notion that language is independent of other aspects of the mind as proposed by Chomsky and other modularity advocates. Moreover, to the extent that these relationships between the linguistic and nonlinguistic domains are found to be mediated by the social interactions in which the individual participates, then an experience-dependent, interactionist position will be supported. In fact, Murphy and Abbeduto (2005) have developed a socially mediated model of language development in fragile X syndrome that attempts to account for the relationships described.

Second, Abbeduto et al. (2003) examined the concurrent relationships among various domains of language and cognitive ability for adolescents and young adults with fragile X or Down syndrome and typically developing children matched to them on nonverbal mental age. In particular, they examined correlations among measures of receptive vocabulary, receptive syntax, and cognitive ability. They found that for all groups the receptive language measures were highly correlated with cognitive ability, which is consistent with the longitudinal findings of Roberts et al. (2001). More importantly, Abbeduto et al. also found that, when cognitive ability was partialled out of the relationships among the receptive language measures, the latter were still significantly correlated for the typically developing children; however, there were fewer significant correlations among receptive language measures for the youth with fragile X syndrome and fewer still for the youth with Down syndrome. Such findings raise the possibility that increased maturity brings with it more integration of the different components of language; or, put differently, development works to reduce modularity. Such a conclusion favors an interactionist rather than modularity position.

Third, several investigators have sought to examine the relative contributions of genetic and environmental variation to the behavioral outcomes of children and adolescents with fragile X syndrome, with several such studies including gross measures of language. Dyer-Friedman, Glaser, Hessl, Johnston, Huffman, Taylor, Wisbeck and Reiss (2002) found that verbal IQs for both boys and girls with fragile X syndrome were predicted by a measure of responsiveness of the home environment, even after controlling for the effects of parental IQ and child FMRP levels. Similarly, Glaser, Hessl, Dyer-Friedman, Johnstone, Wisbeck, Taylor and Reiss (2003) found that variation in adaptive behavior, including in the communication domain, was explained in part by variations in environmental responsiveness for males with fragile X syndrome. Such findings provide support for interactionist accounts of language development.

In summary, the results for fragile X syndrome, like the results for Down syndrome, challenge various tenets of the modularity position. Instead, the findings support the interactionist position in which language learning is seen to be influenced by, and influence, many other domains of development and is highly dependent on experience in a socially responsive and supportive environment.

11. Implications for clinical practice

There remain many gaps in our knowledge about the extent, nature, and causes of the phenotype, including its linguistic dimensions, in fragile X syndrome. Nevertheless, it is possible to derive several implications for current clinical practice. First, it is clear that despite having the linguistic tools to perform at mental age-appropriate levels in communicative interactions, individuals with fragile X syndrome often fail to do so. This suggests that intervention must target not only the acquisition of new vocabulary and syntax, but also strategies for using new and existing forms in socially effective ways. Second, it is clear that there are intimate connections between the development and use of language and other nonlinguistic skills and behaviors. This implies that efforts to improve language and its use must also attempt to impart new cognitive and social-cognitive skills that may be prerequisites for language as well as remove barriers to langue learning and use (e.g., by reducing anxiety and hyperarousal). And finally, it is important to recognize that although there is a typical behavioral phenotype associated with fragile X syndrome, there is considerable individual variability that must be attended to in language assessment and intervention. In other words, clinicians should use their knowledge of the phenotype as a starting point to guide their assessment, while probing for the idiosyncratic strengths, weaknesses, and needs of the individual (Mirrett et al. 2003).

12. Integrating research on Down syndrome and fragile X syndrome

Although there are commonalities in the behavioral phenotypes of Down syndrome and fragile X syndrome, there are, as we have seen, differences as well. These differences include speech intelligibility problems (more severe in Down syndrome), auditory acuity (favoring those with fragile X syndrome), the relative delays of expressive and receptive language (more pronounced in Down syndrome, at least by adolescence), a syntactic deficit relative to nonverbal cognition (more pronounced in Down syndrome). Differences also extend beyond the domain of language to include differences in sociability (favoring Down syndrome), conceptual knowledge of the social world (favoring fragile X syndrome), and the presence of psychopathology and maladaptive behavior (more prevalent in fragile X syndrome). Direct comparisons of the two syndromes as regards language leaning and use may thus provide further insights not only into the mechanisms underlying the emergence of each syndrome's phenotype, but also of language development more generally.

Abbeduto and his colleagues have conducted such direct comparisons and with interesting results. Such comparisons have demonstrated, for example, that although youth with Down or fragile X syndrome are both poor at resolving their comprehension problems relative to mental age-matched typically developing children, the former are especially poor (Abbeduto & Murphy 2004). Additionally, youth with Down syndrome are less inclined to provide scaffolding for their listener's comprehension of referential descriptions when that scaffolding requires producing longer, more complicated utterances (Abbeduto & Murphy 2004). And finally, Abbeduto and colleagues (2003) have demonstrated that youth with Down syndrome acquire receptive vocabulary but not receptive syntax at a similar rate to their age peers with fragile X syndrome. To the extent that these differences in the domain of language are found to be related to differences on nonlinguistic dimensions of the behavioral phenotypes, then we will have further evidence against a modularity position and in favor of an interactionist position. In fact, some such relationships have been established (Abbeduto & Murphy 2004). It is hoped that further comparisons of Down and fragile X syndromes (and other syndromes) will be made in future research. Such comparisons hold promise for both clinical and theoretical work.

Notes

* Preparation of this chapter was supported by NIH grants ROIHD23353, ROIHD24356 and P3OHDD3352.

1. *Series editors' comment*: it is our editorial policy to list all authors at first mention, rather than just the first author and 'et al.'. Although this may lead to textually rather awkward situations, we feel that all authors, especially in groundbreaking work such as the DNA-research cited here, have a right to be mentioned in the text at least once.

The role of language and communication impairments within autism

Morton Ann Gernsbacher, Heather M. Geye
and Susan Ellis Weismer

Delays in language development and impairments in communication ability constitute a defining feature of autism. However, these language and communication impairments can be quite varied, even in classic Autistic Disorder. By current diagnostic definition (ICD-10, World Health Organization 1993; DSM-IV, American Psychiatric Association 1994), these impairments can range from a delay in the development of expressive language to a total lack of expressive language, from problems with initiating or sustaining a conversation to use of stereotyped, repetitive, and idiosyncratic language. In this chapter we first describe the historical interpretation of the basis for the language and communication impairments in autism, beginning with Kanner's (1943) description of his 11 seminal patients and continuing through the 1990s. We then identify an emerging view of the role of language and communication impairments within autism, namely that they overlap, perhaps considerably, with the language and communication impairments observed outside of autism. We then review numerous empirical studies that have demonstrated this overlap. We conclude by offering recommendations for further, necessary empirical investigations and the theoretical implications of those investigations.

1. History of language/communication impairments in autism: Kanner's 11 patients

Communication impairments have been among the defining features of autism since Kanner (1943) first described his eleven seminal patients. The first child, Donald T., arrived at the Harriet Lane Home when he was 5 years, 1 month of age. Before the age of 2, Donald could recite "short poems and even learned the Twenty-third Psalm and twenty-five questions and answers of the Presbyterian Catechism" (Kanner 1943/ reprinted 1985: 11). However, his parents were concerned because "he was not learning to ask questions or to answer questions" (p. 11). During his two-week evaluation, Donald frequently engaged in "verbal rituals" (p. 13) using delayed echolalia by repeating phrases and questions his mother had asked him previously. As an example, when he wanted to get up after his nap, he would ask his mother to say "Don, do you want to get down?" and his mother would repeat the question to him verbatim. Donald would then tell his mother to say "All right" at which point Donald would be able to get up from his nap (p. 13). If his mother did not play her role in these verbal rituals, Donald would throw a temper tantrum. Donald believed in literal, inflexible meanings to words and "he seemed unable to generalize, to transfer an expression to another similar object or situation" (p. 14). By the age of 6;6,[1] his mother reported that "he talks very much more and asks a good many questions. Not often does he voluntarily tell me of happenings at school, but if I ask leading questions, he answers them correctly" (p. 16).

The mother of the second child, Frederick W., reported that "he had said at least two words ('daddy' and 'Dora') before he was 2 years old. From then on, between 2 and 3 years, he would say words that seemed to come as a surprise to himself. He'd say them once and then never repeat them" (p. 18). When Frederick was 4 years old, his mother tried to make him use words to ask for something he wanted or she would not give him the desired object, but he refused to comply. His mother also reported that he had great difficulty with the correct use of personal pronouns. Frederick was seen at the Harriet Lane Home when he was 6 years old. At that time, "when he responded to questions or commands at all, he did so by repeating them echolalia fashion" (p. 19).

Richard M. was brought to Johns Hopkins Hospital at 3;3 because his parents suspected that he was deaf as he did not talk or respond to questions. The intern who admitted Richard observed that "it is difficult to tell definitely whether he hears, but it seems that he does" as he obeyed commands "even when he does not see the speaker and he does not pay attention to conversation going on around him" (p. 20). During his evaluation, he "uttered short staccato forceful sounds – 'Ee! Ee! Ee!' He complied with a spoken and gestural command of his mother to take off his slippers" (p. 21). However, when she asked him a different command without gesture accompanying her speech, he again took off his slippers. At two subsequent visits to Johns Hopkins before his fifth birthday, he failed to display any expressive language gains.

By the time Paul G., the fourth child, was 3 years old, he could recite "not less than thirty-seven songs and various sundry nursery rhymes" (p. 22). During his evaluation, when he was 5 years old, he played with a toy telephone, "singing again and again, 'he wants the telephone"' (p. 23) and while using a pair of scissors to cut a piece of paper into small pieces, he sang over and over, "cutting paper" (p. 23). Paul also engaged in many instances of delayed echolalia, repeating sentences he had heard before, such as "Did you hurt your leg?", "You'll fall off the bicycle and bump your head", and "Don't throw the dog off the balcony" (p. 23). However, while Paul had a large vocabulary and used language frequently, he did not use language as a means to communicate with others. Additionally, like Frederick, he had great difficulty with the correct use of personal pronouns. His mother reported that he had never referred to himself with the first person pronoun. For example, when he wanted candy, he would say, "You want candy."

The prominent psychiatrist father of child five, Barbara K., described his 8-year-old daughter as having had "ordinary vocabulary at 2 years, but always slow at putting words into sentences," having "difficulty with verbal expression," and repeating phrases (Kanner 1943:25). The father reported that the child had previously shown difficulty with the correct use of personal pronouns. During her evaluation when she was 8;3, Barbara was able to comment on a pen on the desk ("Pen like yours at home") and ask for a pencil ("May I take this home?"). She frequently interrupted other conversations and interjected her own irrelevant information (such as "I saw motor transports" and "I saw piggy-back when I went to school").

Child six, Virginia S., like Richard, was at one time suspected to be deaf. However, a psychologist at the state training school for the feebleminded (where Virginia had been a resident since she was 5 years old), observed that just before her 7th birthday, Virginia could respond to sounds, including her name being called. The psychologist reported that "she pays no attention to what is said to her, but quickly comprehends whatever is expected" (p. 27). Some of the other children she roomed with at the state training school reported that when Virginia was 8;9, she was able to produce some single words, including "chocolate," "marshmallow, "mama," and "baby." During an evaluation when Virginia was 11 years old, she occasionally answered "mamma, baby" in response to questions directed at her.

Herbert B., child seven, was also at one time suspected to be deaf because he appeared to pay little attention when others spoke to him and he appeared to make little attempt to speak. According to his physician mother at the time of his referral at 3;2, he had always been quiet. He returned to the clinic two more times (at ages 4;7 and 5;2). Herbert still did not speak, nor did he respond to any speech addressed to him during either of those visits. However, he occasionally produced "inarticulate sounds in a monotonous singsong manner" (p. 30).

Alfred L., the eighth child, was seen at the clinic for the first time at 3;6. At that time, his clinical psychologist mother reported that "language developed slowly; he seemed to have no interest in it. He seldom tells experience. He still confuses pronouns. He never asks questions in the form of questions (with appropriate inflection). Since he talked, there has been a tendency to repeat over and over one word or statement. He almost never says a sentence without repeating it" (p. 30). By the age of 9 years, 1 month, his language was grammatically correct, but included many obsessive questions regarding his current topic of interest (darkness and light). When asked to define words such as balloon and tiger, he was "painstakingly specific in his definitions" (p. 32), yet he was "often confused about the meaning of words" (p. 33).

The mother of child nine, Charles N., described his language at 4;6 as nothing more than a repetition of what had been said to him. Additionally, he did not use personal pronouns correctly, always using the third person rather than the first person when talking about himself. His mother said that he had a good vocabulary, but that he "never initiates conversation, and conversation is limited, extensive only as far as objects go" (p. 34), and Kanner noted that "he never used language as a means of communicating with people" (p. 35).

At the time that, John F., the tenth child, was seen at the clinic for the first time at 2;4, his vocabulary was rather limited. Three months later, his vocabulary "showed remarkable improvement, though his articulation was defective" (p. 36). By the end of his fourth year, "he was capable of forming elaborate and grammatically correct sentences," (p. 36) but his language was full of many examples of both immediate and delayed echolalia. Additionally at this age, he did not use personal pronouns correctly. Unlike Charles (who used the third person personal pronoun), John used the second person personal pronoun when referring to himself. He began using pronouns correctly at 4;6, and by 5;6, "he had a good mastery of the use of pronouns" (p. 37).

The final child, Elaine C., was 7;2 when she was first seen at the clinic. Her parents reported that "she could say four words at the end of her first year, but made no progress in linguistic development for the following four years" (p. 38). Like several of the other children, deafness was suspected and subsequently ruled out. When she finally began to speak at 5 years of age, she started out with "complete though simple sentences" (p. 38). A Boston psychologist who examined Elaine when she was 7 years old stated that she could name a wide variety of objects, but that she "rarely answered a direct question" (p. 39). The psychologist also noted her tendency to repeat contextually irrelevant phrases over and over again, which quite possibly was a display of delayed echolalia. Elaine was observed for three weeks at the Child Study Home of Maryland when she was 7;2. During her evaluation, the doctors noted that her speech was rarely communicative, that her grammar was inflexible, and that she repeated sentences just as she heard them (e.g., she repeated "Want me to draw a spider" rather than saying "I want you to draw a spider," p. 40).

Thus, all of Kanner's (1943) eleven patients exhibited communication impairments, although the impairments varied widely. Over half the children exhibited delayed early language development, and three of the children never developed fluent spoken language. Parents of four of the children reported that at one time they suspected that their child was deaf. Of the eight children who could speak, nearly all displayed examples of immediate or delayed echolalia and impairments in their use of personal pronouns, and several were reported to not use language as a means of communication. Additionally, several of the children displayed literalness in the meanings of their words, and a couple used verbal rituals in their daily conversations.

2. History of the role of language/communication impairments in autism: 1970–1990

Kanner did not attribute the language and communication impairments he observed in his patients to psycholinguistic origins; rather, Kanner viewed these impairments solely as manifestations of the children's social or emotional impairments. Twenty-five years later, the tide turned. In the 1970s, the language and communication impairments found within autism were not only presumed to be psycholinguistic in origin, they were believed to be identical to the language and communication impairments found outside of autism, differing only in their severity. For example, Churchill (1972, as quoted in Bishop 1989: 113) proposed that "there was no qualitative distinction between 'developmental aphasia' and autism, and that they differed only in degree." Wing (1976, as quoted in Bishop 1989: 114) predicted that "if children … could be arranged in an orderly series, starting from the most autistic child at one end and extending to the child who most clearly had nothing but a developmental receptive speech disorder at the other, to say where the dividing line should be drawn would need the judgment of Solomon."

Rutter's early work similarly claimed that some of the communication impairments found in autistic disorder were "almost synonymous with childhood dysphasia." In one study, Bartak, Rutter and Cox (1975) examined 42 children with severe developmental receptive language disorder, 19 of whom were diagnosed with autism (mean age = 7;0), and 23 were diagnosed with developmental language disorder (impaired comprehension and production) without autistic features and referred to as dysphasic (mean age = 8;2). All the children had nonverbal IQs of at least 70. The children's expressive language was measured by the Reynell Developmental Language Scales (Reynell 1969) and through a sample of spontaneous speech from a free play session with the examiner. No significant differences were found in the mean length of utterance between the two groups or in the grammatical complexity of their speech. While both groups showed developmental delay in the production of single words (58% for the autistic group and 65% for the dysphasic group) and phrase speech (89% for the autistic group and 83% for the dysphasic group), the groups did not differ significantly from each other. The groups also did not differ significantly in the production of abnormal or diminished babble as toddlers (42% for the autistic group and 65% for the dysphasic group). Finally, there was no difference between the groups on family history of speech disorder (26% for the autistic group and 26% for the dysphasic group).

Moreover, those children whom Rutter identified in the late 1970s as only language impaired exhibited 20 years later strong autistic behaviors in adulthood (Howlin, Mawhood, & Rutter 2000). In a follow-up study, conducted when the participants were in their early to mid-twenties, the autism group continued to show impairments in stereotyped behavior patterns, social functioning, social relationships, jobs, and independence (Howlin et al. 2000). However, the language impaired group (known previously as the dysphasic group) also displayed impairments in all of these areas. Over half (55%) of the language impaired group were rated as having "intermediate" levels of problem behavior on the Vineland Maladaptive Behavior Domain, and less than half obtained "adequate" scores in any of the three sub-domains on the Vineland Socialization Domain. Additionally, well over half of the language impaired group experienced challenges in establishing spontaneous reciprocal social relationships, over a third had no friends, and two thirds had never had a close sexual relationship. While general ratings of friendship had remained unchanged over time in the autism group, they had deteriorated in over two thirds of the language impaired group. Many of the participants in the language impaired group still lived with their parents, and few had permanent jobs.

The 1980s witnessed the widespread assumption that the sole, or at least primary, deficits of communication in autism were pragmatic in nature (Paul & Cohen 1984, 1985; Lord, Rutter, Goode, Heemsbergen, Jordan, Mawhood, & Schopler 1989). For example, Paul and Cohen (1984) compared eight individuals with autism (mean age = 22.3 years) with eight IQ-matched adults with mental retardation (mean age = 29.5 years). The autism group was significantly inferior to the mental retardation group in the understanding of figurative and comparative language (as measured by the Clinical Evaluation of Language Functions; CELF). When assessed for their request-for-clarification abilities (e.g., Speaker 1 states, "I watched *Dynasty* last night" followed by Speaker 2 asking, "You watched what?"), the participants with autism responded to the contingent queries an average of 93% of the time; however, they were less likely than the mental retardation group to supply the specific constituent requested. Rather, they tended to repeat or revise their utterance "as if they were unable to identify from the query which piece of information needed clarification" (Paul & Cohen 1984: 356). The authors concluded that the deficits in contingent queries displayed by the autism group were due to impairments in "the ability to make the social judgments that dictates the choice of linguistic form in discourse" (p. 356).

Using almost the same participant sample, Paul and Cohen (1985) compared the comprehension of 20 indirect requests, each with varying syntactic complexity, by the group of eight adults with autism (mean age = 22.3 years) and the eight IQ-matched adults with mental retardation (mean age = 27.9 years). In a structured condition the experimenter directly prefaced requests ("I'm going to ask you to color some circles; color them either red or blue according to what I say"), whereas in the pragmatic condition the experimenter made indirect requests during the middle of a conversation. While the performance of the group with mental retardation remained constant across conditions, the performance of the group with autism was significantly better in the structured condition than the pragmatic condition. Paul and Cohen concluded that explicit cues were necessary in order for the autism group to comprehend the speaker's intention.

Lord et al. (1989) examined the reliability of the Autism Diagnostic Observation Schedule (ADOS), a semi-structured, standardized protocol for the observation of social and communicative behavior associated with autism. They compared four groups of 20 children: autistic/mildly retarded (mean age = 13;0) autistic/non-retarded (mean age = 13;0), mentally handicapped (mean age = 13;0), and typically developing (mean age = 12;11). Of the 30 items (including 11 items of social interactions, 10 items of communication/language,

3 items of restricted/stereotyped behavior, and 6 mood/nonspecific abnormal behaviors), only two communication/language items – idiosyncratic language and inappropriate questions and statements – significantly differentiated the two autism groups from the two non-autism groups. Both of these communication/language items are highly pragmatic in nature, providing support for the argument that communication impairments in autism were pragmatic in nature. Indeed, the assumption that deficits of communication in autism were primarily pragmatic in nature was held so strongly during the 1980s that in one study children with autism's omission of the regular past tense and present progressive (compared with their relatively intact usage of the regular third-person and possessive) was interpreted as a sign of pragmatic impairment (Bartolucci, Pierce, & Streiner 1980).

The 1990s continued to embrace the assumption that the primary deficits of communication in autism were pragmatic and went further to attribute the pragmatic deficits to challenges in social-cognition. An example of one of the social-cognitive explanations was the theory of mind hypothesis (Tager-Flusberg 1999). Theory of mind refers to "the ability to attribute mental states, such as desire, knowledge, and belief, to oneself and other people as a means of explaining behavior" (Tager-Flusberg 1999: 326). By 4 years of age, typically developing children are assumed to understand that others may hold beliefs that conflict with reality, known as false beliefs. The conventional test for theory of mind is the false belief test, in which the child is told a story about Sally and Anne. Sally places a marble in a basket and then leaves the room, leaving the marble in the basket. Anne, who is still in the room, then takes the marble from the basket and places it in a box. The child is then asked to predict where Sally will look for the marble when she returns to the room. To answer correctly, the child must disregard his/her knowledge of the actual location of the marble because Sally does not have this information. In several early studies, autistic children were more likely to fail a false belief test than were mental age matched controls. This poorer performance on the false belief test was taken as strong evidence that autistic children were specifically impaired in their ability to interpret human behavior within a "mentalistic framework" (Tager-Flusberg 1999: 326).

However, it has now been demonstrated that linguistic sophistication underlies success on theory of mind tasks. Steele, Joseph and Tager-Flusberg (2003) utilized a longitudinal approach to examine the developmental trajectory of theory of mind abilities in 57 children with autism (mean age = 92 months). Receptive vocabulary, assessed with the Peabody Picture Vocabulary Test (PPVT), and expressive vocabulary, assessed using the Expressive

Vocabulary Test (EVT; Williams 1997) were assessed at an initial visit and at follow-up one year later. Additionally, ten theory of mind tasks, ranging from early (e.g., desire) to advanced (e.g., moral judgment), were administered to all participants. Scores on the PPVT, EVT, and the theory of mind tasks improved significantly between the initial testing and the one-year follow-up. Vocabulary at the initial assessment was significantly correlated with theory of mind scores at the initial assessment ($r = 0.85, p < .01$) and with theory of mind scores at follow-up ($r = 0.87, p < .01$). The authors, therefore, suggested that "language plays a causal role in the development of theory of mind abilities in both normally developing children and children with autism" (p. 465).

Similarly, Happé (1995) reported age-independent correlations between theory of mind scores and scores on the British Peabody Vocabulary Test (BPVS, Dunn, Dunn, Whetton, & Pintilie 1982), and Eisenmajer and Prior (1991) found that both verbal mental age and pragmatic ability were superior among children with autism who passed theory of mind tasks. Tager-Flusberg and Sullivan (1994) also found that PPVT scores correlated with theory of mind performance in children with autism; however, in their study, a stronger correlation with theory of mind tests was found for a sentence comprehension measure of syntactic knowledge (the Sentence Structure subtest on the Clinical Evaluation of Language Fundamentals, CELF, Semel, Wiig, & Secord 1987). More recently, Tager-Flusberg has suggested that acquisition of sentential complements is a core predictor of which children with autism will pass theory of mind tests (Tager-Flusberg 1997, 2000). Tager-Flusberg and Joseph (in press) examined 51 children with autism who were between the ages of 5;4 and 14;2 at the start of a two- year longitudinal study. IPSyn scores, a measure of general syntactic and morphological development (Index of Productive Syntax; Scarborough 1990), explained a significant amount of the variance in Year 2 theory of mind score, especially in the analyses of the concurrent predictors of theory of mind. Specific knowledge of sentential complements accounted for significant additional variance in predicting both concurrent and longitudinal performance on theory of mind tasks.

While some researchers in the 1990s were attributing the pragmatic deficits observed in autism to a lack of a theory of mind, others were attributing them to other social-cognitive constructs. For example, Mundy, Sigman and Kasari (1990), attributed the pragmatic deficits to a deficit or delay in joint attention. In one study, fifteen autistic children (mean age = 45 months) were matched with 15 children on mental age (mean age = 29 months), and 15 children on language age (mean age = 25 months). Nonverbal communication skills were assessed twice (initially and at follow-up 13 months later) with an abridged form of the Early Social-Communication Scales (ESCS; Seibert, Hogan, & Mundy 1982), which examines the social behavior, joint attention, and requesting behavior of children. The autistic children displayed fewer joint attention behaviors than both of the comparison groups. Language development was assessed initially and then at follow-up 13 months later using the Reynell Developmental Language Scales. ESCS scores from the first testing session were correlated with the Reynell language age estimates from the follow-up testing. Joint attention was a significant predictor of language development in the autistic group ($r = 0.61, p < .05$).

However, other studies have found that joint attention is unrelated to language development within children with autism. For example, Morgan, Maybery and Durkin (2003) examined 21 children with autism (mean age = 54 months) and 21 typically developing children (mean age = 55 months) on three measures of joint attention. Although the children with autism demonstrated significantly lower rates of joint attention as measured by each of the three tasks, vocabulary development (as measured by the PPVT) was neither correlated with joint attention within the autism group nor a mediator of the difference between the two participant groups on the measures of joint attention. In other words, joint attention and language development were independent (see also Loveland & Landry 1986; Stone & Yoder 2001). Gernsbacher, Sauer, Geye, O'Reilly and Goldsmith (submitted) reported a case study of child with autism (birth to 8;0) who has never shown traditional indicators of joint attention (pointing, showing, and tripartite gaze), but who nonetheless has age-advanced receptive and non-speech expressive language.

3. Emerging view of the role of language/communication impairments within autism

An emerging view of the role of language and communication impairments within autism is that they overlap, perhaps considerably, with the language and communication impairments observed outside of autism. For example, there is empirical evidence for behavioral overlap between the language and communication challenges observed in autism and those observed in (i) Specific Language Impairment (SLI, which is impaired language in the face of otherwise typical development; Baltaxe & D'Anglia 1996; Bishop & Norbury 2002; Joseph, Tager-Flusberg, & Lord 2002; Kjelgaard & Tager-Flusberg 2001; Paul, Fischer, & Cohen 1988), (ii) Pragmatic Language Impairment (which is impaired use of pragmatic language in children whose non-language behaviors fall outside the autism spectrum; Bishop & Norbury 2002; Botting & Conti-Ramsden 2003); (iii) Landau-Kleffner Syndrome (Nass, Gross, & Devinsky 1998; Rossi, Parmeggiani, Posar, Scaduto, Chiodo, & Vatti 1999; Shinnar, Rapin, Arnold, Tuchman, Shulman, Ballanan-Gill, Maw, Deuel, & Volkmar 2001); and (iv) early language delay (as manifested by vocabulary development, gestural use, and comprehension; Charman, Drew, Baird, & Baird 2003a). Each of these arenas of overlap will be reviewed briefly below.

4. The overlap between autism and Specific Language Impairment (SLI)

Baltaxe and D'Angiola (1996) compared the use of referencing strategies (pronominal, demonstrative, and comparative) produced in a one-hour free play session with an experimenter in three groups of children matched for sex, social class, and language age (including MLU in morphemes, receptive vocabulary age on PPVT-R, and language comprehension on the Test of Auditory Comprehension of Language; TACL). The three groups comprised 10 children with autism (mean age = 93 months), eight with SLI (mean age = 92 months), and eight with typical language development (mean age = 42 months). All three groups used personal pronouns most frequently, followed by demonstrative reference, and then comparative reference. However, both the autism and the SLI groups produced significantly fewer correct examples of all types of referencing categories, and the autism and SLI groups did not differ significantly from each other. The typically developing group used first person pronouns significantly more than either the autism or SLI groups, and the amount of first person pronoun usage did not differ significantly between the autism and SLI groups.

During later childhood some children originally diagnosed with SLI show autistic symptoms in non-language domains (Bishop & Norbury 2002). A third of SLI children (including those with SLI-T and PLI) exhibited abnormal imagination/creativity and over- activity/agitation on the ADOS-G and approximately 20% exhibited abnormal excessive interest in objects and unusual sensory interest on the ADOS-G (Bishop & Norbury 2002).

Joseph, Tager-Flusberg and Lord (2002) examined the verbal and nonverbal abilities in 120 children with autism using the Differential Ability Scales (DAS) and the Autism Diagnostic Observation Schedule. The Preschool DAS was administered to 73 children between the ages of 3;8 and 6;11 (mean age = 5;5), and the School-Age DAS was administered to 47 children between 7;0 and 13;11 (mean age = 8;11). Almost half the children administered the

Preschool DAS (48%) and a third of the children administered the School-Age DAS (34%) exhibited substantially lower verbal IQ than nonverbal IQ scores, meeting diagnostic criteria for SLI.

Kjelgaard and Tager-Flusberg (2001) examined the phonological, lexical, and higher order language abilities in 89 children with autism (mean age = 88 months) using a battery of tests (including the Goldman-Fristoe Test of Articulation, which measured productive phonology for consonants in English; the PPVT-III; the EVT, which measures expressive vocabulary; the CELF, which measures morphology, syntax, semantics, and working memory; and repetition of nonsense words, which assesses the ability to reproduce words). Using methodology commonly used in SLI research, the researchers divided the 82 children who completed the PPVT into three groups: the normal group (standard PPVT scores of $\geq$ to 85; n = 22), the borderline group (standard PPVT scores between 70 and 84; n = 10) and the impaired group (standard PPVT scores below 70; n = 50). Fourteen children (28%) in the impaired language group had nonverbal IQ scores above 70, and nine children in the normal language group (41%) had nonverbal IQs in the borderline to mentally retarded range. Thus, the researchers concluded that language skills "can be independent of IQ in autism" (p. 301). Furthermore, the children's overall vocabulary scores, PPVT ($M = 85.57$) and EVT ($M = 84.9$), were greater than their knowledge of syntax and semantics, CELF Total $M = 72.3$, CELF-Receptive $M = 70.9$, CELF-Expressive $M = 74.9$), which, the researchers argued, is similar to the profile of abilities found in children with SLI. Thus, Kjelgaard and Tager-Flusberg (2001) concluded that their "profile analysis may be taken as evidence for theoretically significant overlap between SLI and autism" (p. 304).

Paul et al. (1988) examined the sentence comprehension strategies in six children with autism (mean age = 6.5 years), seven language impaired (LI) children (mean age = 4.8 years), eight typically developing children matched on receptive language age (mean age = 34.8 months), and eight typically developing children matched on nonverbal mental age (mean age = 43.4 months). A speech-language pathologist tested the children individually on 24 test sentences that the children were instructed to act out. Half the sentences were in active voice, and half were in passive voice. Within each voice set, there were three subsets: probable (e.g., the girl carries the baby), neutral (e.g., the truck pushes the car), and improbable (e.g., the baby carries the girl) sentences. While the autism and the LI children produced fewer correct responses for both the improbable active (autism $M = 1.5$ out of 4, LI $M = 1.6$ out of 4) and passive (autism $M = 0.7$ out of 4, LI $M = 0.4$ out of 4) voice sentences than the typically developing 3-year-olds (active $M = 3.3$; passive $M = 2.1$), the performance between the autism and LI groups did not differ significantly. The authors concluded that the autism and LI children "who are at similar stages of language and cognitive development appear to perform more similarly than might be expected on this comprehension task" (p. 678).

Speculation has even arisen from quantitative genetics of a locus of susceptibility common to autism and SLI (O'Brien, Zhang, Nishimura, Tomblin, & Murray 2003; Warburton, Baird, Chen, Morris, Jacobs, Hodgson, & Docherty 2000, but see Newbury & Monaco 2002); such speculation is supported by behavioral genetic data demonstrating an increased risk of autism to siblings of children with SLI (Tomblin, Hafeman, & O'Brien 2003) and an increased risk of SLI to siblings of children with autism (Fombonne, Bolton, Prior, Jordan, & Rutter 1997; Folstein, Santangelo, Gilman, Piven, Landa, Lainhart, Hein, & Wzorek 1999). Tomblin et al. (2003) assessed the autistic behaviors of 522 biological (full or half) siblings of 158 children with SLI and 132 children with normal language abilities on the Autism Behavior Checklist, the Autism Diagnostic Interview-Revised, and the Autism Diagnostic Observation Schedule. Ten siblings were identified as being at risk for autism based on scores from the Autism Behavior Checklist ($\geq$ 57), and six of those 10 were siblings of SLI children. Additionally, the parents of three siblings of SLI children reported their children had received an autism diagnosis. Although not significant, the risk for autism was greater in the siblings of children with SLI than siblings of children with normal language abilities. In addition, when the language proficiency of the probands (*z*-scores of at or below –1.25 SD in 2 of 5 areas of language function while in kindergarten) was taken into account, risk for autism was found only in siblings with probands with poor spoken language.

Fombonne et al. (1997) inquired about the history of any developmental disorders of language, articulation, speech, reading or spelling, and abnormalities of conversational abilities in the first-degree relatives of 99 autism probands (198 parents with mean age = 50;0 and 153 siblings with mean age = 20;4) and 36 Down syndrome controls (72 parents with mean age = 52;1 and 65 siblings with mean age = 25;2). Nearly a quarter of the parents and siblings of the autistic probands had delayed language onset or reading compared to less than 10% of the parents and siblings of the controls. Folstein et al. (1999) also inquired about the history of any developmental disorders of language, articulation, speech, reading or spelling in the parents (n = 166, mean age = 45;6) and siblings (n = 87, mean age = 18;9) of 90 autistic probands and in the parents (n = 75, mean age = 44;8) and siblings (n = 64, mean age = 18;5) of 40 Down Syndrome controls. Twenty-six percent of the autistic parents reported a history of probable or definite language delay, articulation defects, trouble learning to read, or trouble spelling compared to only 11% of the parents of the controls ($c^2 = 6.73$, $p < .01$); fathers more likely than mothers to report these impairments. Interestingly, the autism-parents without any early language-related impairments achieved higher Verbal IQ scores than those achieved by the entire group of autism-parents. A similar relationship was found in the siblings of children with autism, with the siblings without any early language-related impairments achieving higher scores on the Full Scale IQ, Verbal IQ, the Kaufman Reading Comprehension test, and the Schonell spelling test than the siblings with early language-related impairments.

5. The overlap between autism and pragmatic language impairment

Bishop and Norbury (2002; study 1) assessed 13 children with pragmatic language impairment (PLI; NVIQ of 80 or above and pragmatic composite score on the Children's Communication Checklist below 133; mean age = 8;3) and eight children with typical SLI (SLI-T; NVIQ of 80 or above, pragmatic composite score on the Children's Communication Checklist above 132 and score on a standardized language test at least 1 SD below the normative mean; mean age = 9;2) on three commonly used autism assessments (the Autism Diagnostic Interview-Revised and the Social Communication Questionnaire, which were administered to the parents, and the Autism Diagnostic Observation Schedule – Generic, which was administered to the children). On the Autism Diagnostic Interview, six children with PLI (46%) and two children with SLI-T (25%) had scores that were above threshold for autistic disorder. Two additional PLI children (15%) and four additional SLI-T children (50%) scored above threshold on two of the three domains, meeting criteria for Pervasive Developmental Disorder-Not Otherwise Specified (PDD-NOS). On the Social Communication Questionnaire, five PLI children (39%) and two SLI-T children (25%) met criteria for autistic disorder, while an additional two PLI children (15%) and three SLI-T children (38%) met criteria for PDD-NOS. On the Autism Diagnostic Observation Schedule, six children with PLI (46%) and one child with SLI-T (13%) met criteria for autistic disorder, while and two additional PLI children (15%) and one additional SLI-T child (13%) met criteria for PDD-NOS. Thus, around 40% of the children with PLI met criteria for autistic disorder, and another 15% met criteria for PDD-NOS. Bishop and Norbury (2002) argued that these data demonstrated that "many language-impaired children have some pragmatic abnormalities, and some have other features of autism" (p. 922).

Bishop and Norbury (2002; study 2) assessed 18 children with PLI (mean age = 9.2 years), 11 children with SLI-T (mean age = 9.45 years), six children with autism (mean age = 9.44 years), and 18 typically developing children (mean age = 8.56 years) on the Social Communication Questionnaire and the Autism Diagnostic Observation Schedule. On the Social Communication Questionnaire, five children with PLI (28%), four children with autism (67%), and one child with SLI-T (9%) met criteria for Autistic Disorder; an additional four children with PLI (22%), two children with SLI-T (18%), and one child with autism (17%) met criteria for PDD-NOS. On the Autism Diagnostic Observation Schedule, three children with PLI (17%) and three children with autism (50%) met criteria Autistic Disorder, and an additional three children with PLI (17%), one child with autism (17%), and one child with SLI-T (9%) met criteria for PDD-NOS. Botting and Conti-Ramsden (2003) compared 13 children with autism (mean age = 10;10), 25 PLI children (mean age = 11;3), and 29 SLI-T children (mean age = 10;10) on a series of psycholinguistic tests, including the Children's Non-Word Repetition (CNRep), the Past Tense Task (PTT), and the CELF Recalling Sentences subtest, which have previously been effective descriptors of SLI. The children with autism did not differ significantly from the children with PLI on their performance on any of the three psycholinguistic measures.

6. The overlap between autism and Asperger's disorder

Although by diagnostic definition, Asperger's Disorder is not characterized by an early history of language delay or by a set of symptoms describing communication impairments, several studies have shown that children and adults diagnosed with Asperger's Disorder nonetheless demonstrate language and communication impairments, often quite similar to those found in Autistic Disorder. For example, Howlin (2003) examined the current linguistic functioning of 34 adults with autism with a history of childhood speech delay (assigned to the Autistic Disorder group; mean age = 27.6 years) and 42 adults with autism without a history of childhood speech delay (assigned to the Asperger's Disorder group; mean age = 26.1 years). The two groups were matched for age and nonverbal IQ. Group assignment was based on developmental speech delay as defined by two items from the ADI-R (i.e., no single word speech by 24 months of age and/or no phrase speech by 3 years of age). Current day receptive vocabulary was assessed using the British Picture Vocabulary Scale (BPVS; Dunn, Dunn, Whetton, & Burley 1997; Dunn et al. 1982), and current day productive vocabulary was assessed with the Expressive One Word Picture Vocabulary Test (EOWPVT; Gardner 1982). Even though the mean chronological age of the Asperger's group was 26.1 years, their age equivalent scores were considerably lower on both the BPVS ($M = 16.09$ years, $SD = 4.17$) and the EOWPVT ($M = 16.60$ years, $SD = 2.63$). Indeed, 57% of the Asperger's group scored below ceiling (18 years) on the BPVS, and 62% scored below ceiling (19 years) on the EOWPVT.

Mayes and Calhoun (2001) compared the current expressive language of 23 children with autism with a history of speech delay (Autistic Disorder) and 24 children with autism without a history of speech delay (Asperger's Disorder). All the children had normal nonverbal intelligence (NVIQs ranged from 80 to 143), and the mean age across groups was 6.1 years. The children's spontaneous conversation were analyzed, and their speech was examined for the presence of 11 atypical speech patterns (including abnormal voice quality/modulation, screeching or making other odd noises, repetitive vocalizations, idiosyncratic jargon, echolalia, idiosyncratic speech, perseverative speech, sporadic and infrequent speech, rote phrases uttered out of context, nonsensical speech, and improper use of pronouns). All the children in the Asperger's Disorder group met DSM-IV Autistic Disorder diagnostic criteria for impairments in communication, either displaying difficulty in initiating or sustaining a conversation or stereotyped and repetitive or idiosyncratic language, and in some cases displaying both symptoms. All except one child in the Asperger's Disorder group displayed one or more of the atypical speech patterns.

Eisenmajer, Prior, Leekam, Wing, Ong, Gould and Welham (1998) compared 46 children with autism (mean age = 11.69 years) whose early language development was delayed and 62 children with autism (mean age = 11.6 years) whose early language development was not delayed. ICD-10 and DSM-IV behavioral criteria were used to assess both group's current day autistic symptomology. Children with autism with a history of early language delay (no single words before 24 months and no use of phrases by 36 months) did not differ in current day autistic symptomotology from children with autism without a history of early language delay; however, the two groups did differ in their current day language skill. Thus, it was the language skill and not the autistic symtomotology that distinguished the two groups.

Finally, Miller and Ozonoff (1997) examined the four children presented in Asperger's seminal 1944 paper. They used DSM-IV criteria for Autistic Disorder to determine whether Asperger's children would receive a current day diagnosis of Autistic Disorder. Three of the four children, Fritz, Harro, and Ernst, each displayed three of the communication impairments listed under the diagnostic criteria for Autistic Disorder, including impaired ability to initiate/sustain conversations, stereotyped, repetitive, or idiosyncratic language, and social play below developmental level. The fourth child, Hellmuth, displayed stereotyped, repetitive, or idiosyncratic language, and social play below developmental level. Miller and Ozonoff also identified the children's impairments in social interactions and restricted behaviors and interests. When all three domains were taken into account, seven professionals (4 child psychiatrists, 1 educational psychologist, and 2 doctoral-level special educators) rated all four of the children described by Asperger as meeting DSM-IV criteria for Autistic Disorder rather than Asperger's Disorder.

7. The overlap between autism and Landau-Kleffner syndrome

Landau-Kleffner Syndrome (LKS, a.k.a. acquired epileptiform aphasia, AEA) is characterized by the profound deterioration of previously acquired receptive and expressive language abilities, usually between 3 and 7 years of age, in association with either clinical seizures or epileptiform electroencephalographic abnormalities. Nass et al. (1998) retrospectively reviewed the charts of children admitted to the Comprehensive Epilepsy Unit at New York University Medical Center between September 1993 and January 1996. Forty-two pediatric patients with a history of language, cognitive, social, and/or behavioral deterioration were selected for further examination. The mean age of evaluation was 5;6. Five were identified with epileptiform discharges in the occipital region and were eliminated from further study. None of the remaining children met strict criteria for LKS. Based on Tuchman's (1997) criteria, the remaining 37 were classified as four with autistic regression, 19 with autistic epileptiform regression, 13 with autism, and one with disintegrative epileptiform regression.

Rossi et al. (1999) observed 11 patients with LKS from a mean age at first observation of 5;7 through a mean age at last observation of 13;6. Autistic-like behavior was present at the first observation in four of the 11 children (36%). At the last observation, autistic-like behavior was still present in two of the children (18%). Shinnar et al. (2001) prospectively identified 177 children (145 males, 32 females) with language regression. Of the 177 children with language regression, 155 had received an autism diagnosis. Children whose language regressed before 36 months had a higher probability of an eventual autism diagnosis (144 of 158 children; 91%) than children whose language regressed at 36 months or later (11 of 19; 58%). Additionally, an eventual autism diagnosis was more common in males (90%) with regressed language than in females (75%). Thirty-two children had a history of seizures. Twenty-two of the children with seizures (69%) also received an autism diagnosis. Seizures were more common in children whose language regressed after 36 months (10 of 19; 53%) than children whose language regressed before 36 months (22 of 158; 14%).

8. The overlap between autism and specific language delay

With the exception of language regression, the recommended early markers – "red flags" – for autism and for specific language delay without autism are synonymous: "no single words by 18 months" and "no two word spontaneous (non-echoed) phrases by 24 months" (Baird, Cass, & Slonims 2003; Filipek, Accardo, Baranek, Cook, Dawson, Gordon, Gravel, Johnson, Kallen, Levy, Minshew, Prizant, Rapin, Rogers, Stone, Teplin, Tuchman, & Volkmar 1999). However, very few studies have examined the early language development of children with autism, and none has compared the early language development of children with autism with that of children with specific language delay. Charman et al. (2003a) compared the early language development of children with autism to the MacArthur Communicative Development Inventory (CDI-Infant form) norms. While nearly all 1-year-old typically developing children respond to their name, to 'no,' and to 'there's mommy/daddy' (Fenson, Resznick, Thal, Bates, Hartung, Pethick, Pethick, & Reilly 1993), only 50% of the children with autism under 2 years of age responded to their name, only 70% responded to 'no,' and only 30% responded to 'there's mommy/daddy.' By 1;4, approximately 90% of typically developing children imitate words (Fenson et al. 1993), but only 30% of the children with autism under 2 years of age imitated words. Additionally, nearly 75% of typically developing children at 1;4 name or label objects (Fenson et al. 1993), but only 15% of the children with autism under 2 years of age named or labeled objects. Finally, while the average number of words produced by typically developing children at 1;4 is 31 words, the mean number of words produced by the children with autism under the age of 2 years was only 7 words.

9. Future directions and recommendations

As previously mentioned, very few studies have looked at language development in very young children with autism; the few studies that have were focused on social cognition constructs (e.g., Charman, Baron-Cohen, Swettenham, Baird, Drew, & Cox 2003b) rather than assessing a broad selection of language behaviors. We suggest that it is imperative to investigate communication and language development as early as possible. Consider an analogy from Williams syndrome: Toddlers with Williams syndrome perform relatively poorly on a language task but relatively well on a numerosity task; adults with Williams syndrome show just the opposite pattern (Paterson, Brown, Gsîdl, Johnson, & Karmiloff-Smith 1999). Thus, it could be injudicious to assume that outcomes observed in older children or adults characterize the starting states in early development. Thus, what are needed are relatively large-scale longitudinal studies, but unfortunately all existing longitudinal language-autism studies have very small samples (Tager-Flusberg, Calkins, Nolin, Baumberger, Anderson, & Chadwick-Dias 1990), were case studies (Cunningham 1966), or the study's duration was quite brief (e.g., one year in Mundy et al. 1990). We echo Nordin and Gillberg's (1998) plea for more prospective, longitudinal studies with ASD children. Even more rare than longitudinal studies are studies of young children with autism using psycholinguistic methodologies, even though such techniques have become commonplace in the study of non-autistic children with language impairment (Edwards & Lahey 1996; Gathercole & Baddeley 1990; Stark & Montgomery 1995).

Most strikingly, to date there have been no comparisons between the early language development of young children with autism and the early language development of young children who are delayed in their language development but do not exhibit autistic behaviors. We recommend comparisons examining early lexical and grammatical development, the mechanisms and patterns of early word learning and vocabulary development, the relationship between lexical and grammatical development, and the relation between language level and verbal repetition behavior. We recommend investigating early lexical development because the mechanisms that support word learning have provided a rich basis of inquiry in typically developing populations (Bauer, Goldfield, & Reznick 2002; Dromi 1999; Hoff & Naigles 2002; Markson & Bloom 2001). Of particular interest is the process of 'fast mapping,' which putatively enables young children to quickly construct lexical representations for unfamiliar words given minimal exposure and has been hypothesized to account for rapid gains in vocabulary. Fast mapping has been examined in young children with typical language development (Behrend, Scofield, & Kleinknecht 2001; Heibeck & Markman 1987; Jaswal & Markman 2001; Wilkinson & Mazzitelli 2003), as well as children with Down syndrome (Chapman, Kay-Raining Bird, & Schwartz 1990), Williams syndrome (Stevens & Karmiloff-Smith 1997) and specific language impairment (Dollaghan 1987; Ellis Weismer & Hesketh 1996, 1998; Eyer, Leonard, Bedore, McGregor, Anderson, & Viescas 2002; Rice, Buhr, & Nemeth 1990). However, fast mapping has not been examined in young children with autism and very little is known about the early word learning processes that support lexical development in this population.

Early grammatical development is of importance because it is posited to depend on lexical development, such that advances in grammar occur only after vocabulary has reached a critical mass (Bates & Goodman 2001; Marchman & Bates 1994). The link between lexical and grammatical skills in typical and atypical development is well documented (Dionne, Dale, Boivin, & Plomin 2003; Maitel, Dromi, Sagi, & Bornstein 2000; Throdardottir, Ellis Weismer, & Evans 2002); however, little is known about this link in autism.

Finally, we recommend investigating verbal repetitions in the language use of young children with and without autism. Verbal repetition can sometimes be a prominent feature of some autistic children's discourse during some stages of their language development; however, the frequently made claim that 75% of all verbal individuals with autism engage often in verbal repetition is most likely a misrepresentation. That 75% figure can be traced to only one empirical study, which was conducted almost four decades ago with children diagnosed with infantile psychosis (Rutter, Greenfield, & Lockyer 1967). While it is true that 75% of the 34 children examined in that study exhibited verbal repetition at some point in their development, there was great variability in the pattern and frequency of the verbal repetition, and for the majority of the children, verbal repetition was not a continuing characteristic in later development (see also Wing 1971). Verbal repetition has been suggested to serve certain communicative functions (Prizant 1983; Prizant & Rydell 1993; Rydell & Mirenda 1994), and verbal repetition has been speculated to reflect lower receptive language skills than would be expected from the child's expressive language skills (Roberts 1989). Thus, an investigation of the verbal repetition exhibited by young children with and without autism is crucial for understanding verbal repetition phenomena.

Examining the early language development of children with autism is of theoretical and practical significance. Of specific theoretical significance are the empirical tests of fundamental language development hypotheses, such as the critical mass hypothesis and the nature of the link between lexical and grammatical development in young children with autism. Of more general theoretical significance is whether the language delays and deficits observed in autism should be considered a unique phenomenon, or whether they overlap with other language and communication disorders. We can refer to these two possibilities as the distinct category account and the dimensional account. The dimensional versus categorical nature of psychopathological conditions such as social anhedonia, depression, and dissociation has been addressed in prior research (Blanchard, Gangestad, Brown, & Horan 2000; Ruscio & Ruscio 2000; Waller, Putnam, & Carlson 1996). In the domain of language disorders, results from an investigation by Whitehurst and Fischel (2000) have been interpreted as indicating the presence of a natural category ('taxon') for dyslexia within a large sample of school-age children. In contrast, recent studies have not provided empirical evidence for a natural category of specific language impairment in large samples of preschool or school age children (SLI; Dollaghan in press; Zhang & Tomblin in preparation). The research focused on dyslexia and SLI has examined distributions of phenomena associated with conditions involving specific deficits relative to normal range reading and spoken language performance. We recommend exploring the overlap in the phenomena associated with language delays in young children with autism and late talkers without autism.

Although the phrasing of the DSM-IV diagnostic criteria (i.e., the use of the term "qualitative impairments") suggests that the language and communication impairments observed in Autistic Disorder and PDD-NOS compose a distinct category, little empirical evidence has directly assessed this assumption. Further research aimed at testing the language distinct account versus the language dimensional account should provide important implications about phenotypic markers (as suggested by Dawson, Webb, Schellenberg, Dager, Friedman, Aylward, & Richards 2002) and by extension, recommended treatment.

Language acquisition in children with a cochlear implant

Karen Schauwers, Steven Gillis and Paul Govaerts

1. Introduction

Children born deaf, or deafened at an early age, with a total or near-total sensorineural hearing loss (i.e. characterized by a malfunctioning cochlea) are unable to acquire language through audition and depend on a visual mode of communication (sign language, lip-reading, or written language). More specifically, it is accepted that a child with a hearing loss in excess of 60 dBHL will not develop good spoken language skills, because normal conversational speech sounds are presented in the 40 dB – 60 dB range. Early amplification by means of hearing aids is helpful for hearing impaired children, but for some children conventional hearing aids provide little or no benefit because their hearing loss is so severe that amplification does not reach the area of the speech spectrum.

A useful categorization of these profoundly hearing impaired children has been introduced by Osberger, Maso and Sam (1993), who divided them into three groups based on unaided and aided hearing thresholds at 500, 1000, and 2000 Hz. *Gold* hearing aid users have unaided pure-tone hearing levels of 90 to 100 dBHL and aided thresholds between 30 and 55 dBHL. In many but not all cases, these Gold hearing aid users will acquire speech and spoken language. *Silver* hearing aid users have unaided thresholds of 101 to 110 dBHL and aided thresholds greater than 55 dBHL. They receive few spectral cues and rely heavily on timing aspects of speech. *Bronze* hearing aid users have unaided thresholds greater than 110 dBHL, which is suggestive of vibrotactile rather than auditory sensation, and these children receive negligible benefit from conventional hearing aids.

For the Silver and Bronze hearing aid users, cochlear implants (CI) can provide access to the auditory information that is essential for spoken language development. A cochlear implant is an electronic device that functions as a sensory aid, converting mechanical sound energy into a coded electrical stimulus that directly stimulates the remaining auditory nerve fibers, bypassing damaged or missing hair cells of the cochlea. Part of the CI is surgically implanted into the cochlea and the mastoid, and the remaining part is worn externally. The external components consist of a microphone, a signal processor, and a transmitter coil. The microphone receives acoustic signals and converts them into an analog electrical signal that is sent to the processor, which modifies the signal into an electrical or digital pattern that is transmitted to the internal part by means of the two coils (the external transmitter coil and the internal receiver coil). The internal part then stimulates the electrodes in the cochlea. The electrodes are thus able to deliver electrical stimulation to excite the cochlear neurons of the auditory nerve. Some 4 weeks after surgery, the initial tuning session of the CI takes place, which is often called "switch-on". In this session, the external parts of the device are programmed and rehabilitation can be started.

In the early days of pediatric implantation, candidacy requirements included an unaided pure-tone average (PTA) of 100 dBHL or more (i.e. Silver and Bronze hearing aid users), aided thresholds of 60 dBHL or worse, and absence of open-set speech discrimination and word recognition with well-fitted hearing aids. Recently, profoundly hearing impaired children with hearing losses of 90 dBHL or sometimes even better also have been considered potential candidates for cochlear implantation. The final decision about their eligibility depends largely upon their performance after prolonged hearing aid use and their ability to discriminate speech sounds.

Most implant users improve to hearing thresholds in the 20 to 40 dBHL range across all frequencies with their device, which corresponds to a mild hearing loss. This means that the implant enables detection of virtually all conversational sounds and provides a hearing sensitivity and functioning which is superior to that obtained with conventional hearing aids. A sensorineural hearing loss is not only characterized by an elevated threshold on pure-tone audiometry, but also by a lower frequency resolution. A good frequency resolving power of the cochlea, however, is essential for normal speech and language development, and lack of it is the key problem in hearing impairment. Hearing impaired people not only fail to hear many sounds, but if they hear them, they often fail to discriminate them. Conventional hearing aids unfortunately only amplify the sound, and don't improve the frequency discrimination. Frequently, the hearing impaired patient reports to hear sound better with a hearing aid, without necessarily better understanding the words. Cochlear implants in contrast not only amplify the sound, but they also aim at a (partial) restoration of the frequency resolution of the cochlea. This is the major advantage of a CI over a hearing aid in cases where the hearing loss is severe to profound and the cochlear tuning becomes deficient.

Detailed studies of the speech and language development of children using CI are just emerging. Initially, the primary function of a CI was to improve the speech perception abilities. As a consequence, research on the benefits of the implant has focused mainly on speech perception, and these studies revealed a continuous improvement of auditory perceptual skills in CI children after implantation (Osberger, Miyamoto, Zimmerman-Phillips, Kemink, Stroer, Firszt, & Novak 1991a; Waltzman, Cohen, Gomolin, Shapiro, Ozdamar, & Hoffman 1994; Snik, Vermeulen, Geelen, Brokx, & van der Broek 1997; Tyler, Fryauf-Bertschy, Kelsay, Gantz, Woodworth, & Parkinson 1997; Waltzman, Cohen, Gomolin, Green, Shapiro, Hoffman, & Roland 1997; Illg, von der Haar-Heise, Goldring, Lesinski-Schiedat, Battmer, & Lenarz 1999; Lenarz, Lesinski-Schiedat, von der Haar-Heise, Illg, Bertram, & Battmer 1999; Govaerts, De Beukelaer, Daemers, De Ceulaer, Yperman, Somers, Schatteman, & Offeciers 2002 and others). Many of these data demonstrate the ability of congenitally or prelingually deaf children to achieve significant and usable open-set speech perception following cochlear implantation at a young age. The increasing belief that cochlear implants also provide feedback to monitor one's own speech, incited a number of investigations in the last decade examining the speech and language production of prelingually deafened CI users.

In this chapter, we will focus on speech and language acquisition of CI children. The major results will be summarized in terms of different linguistic domains: prelexical babbling, phonology, intelligibility, vocabulary, morphosyntaxis, and pragmatics. The typical child reported on in these relevant papers is a prelingually deafened child, being implanted between 3 and 5 years of age and wearing the implant for 2–3 years. Most of the studies selected English-learning children as subjects. If another language is investigated, this will be stated in the text. In addition, an important part of this chapter will be dedicated to the possible factors affecting the language outcomes in CI children. Although a consensus seems to exist on the benefit of CI in children, the outcomes still seem to vary to a great extend. A number of alleged contributing factors will be discussed, including the age at implantation, educational approaches, and the length of CI experience.

2. Comments on methodology in CI studies

Speech and language research in prelingually deafened CI children belongs to a relatively new scientific field and numerous difficulties exist that make the interpretation of data problematic.

The principal difficulty is that CI children constitute a very heterogeneous group with very different audiological and educational characteristics like the age at onset of deafness, the age at implantation, and the communication mode. Also, the individual history of each child may be very different from others. This relates to the age at fitting of conventional hearing aids (before receiving the CI), the type of deafness (i.e. congenitally, prelingually, or postlingually), the amount and type of speech-language therapy before and/or after implantation, the level of sign language ability before and after implantation, etc. All these factors are thought to influence the speech and language development and, unfortunately, they are often poorly defined or even lacking.

It was not until recently that the FDA (i.e. Food and Drug Administration in the USA) approved cochlear implantation below the age of 2 years. As a consequence, the majority of the studies published so far about language acquisition in CI children showed results of deaf children implanted at a mean age between 3 and 5 years. To date this is considered to be "late", since the age at implantation has dropped to below 2 years and in some countries even below 1 year of age. As some studies seem to suggest that receiving an implant before the age of two may lead to greater and faster improvements in speech perception and production than implantation later in childhood (Waltzman & Cohen 1998), further research is needed as younger CI candidates become available.

Another factor that renders the interpretation of results difficult is the fact that CI technology is improving with time. Thus, over time, findings may become obsolete simply because they relate to technology that is no longer in use (like certain types of implants or of speech coding strategies).

Finally, the study of a child in development requires a longitudinal and comparative study design. Unfortunately, longitudinal cohort studies are very time-consuming. This is probably the main reason why the majority of CI investigations are either cross-sectional, or longitudinal over only a short period of time, or longitudinal with too long intervals, or longitudinal case studies. In addition, a matched control group is frequently lacking. The absence of proper longitudinal cohort studies is very problematic.

3. Effectiveness of CI: General measures

Before discussing CI studies in which specific sub-domains of language are considered, the development of language in general in groups of deaf children with a CI will be described. Research focusing on language acquisition frequently use a variety of formal language tests, like the Reynell Developmental Language Scales (RDLS), the Clinical Evaluation of Language Fundamentals (CELF), or the Grammatical Analysis of Elicited Language (GAEL) to evaluate receptive and expressive language skills before and after implantation. Data analysis relies mainly on three quantitative variables: *language age, language quotient*, and the *rate of language change*. For example, a language age (or age-equivalent) score of 36 months implies that the CI child has the language skills equivalent to that of a normally developing child of 3 years old. The language quotient is then calculated by dividing the language age by the chronological age. In order to determine whether there is a significant gain in language age over time, the rate of improvement is calculated by dividing the change in age-equivalent score over time by the change in chronological age over the same time period. A rate of 1.00 represents the "normal" rate of language development, i.e. an equal change of language age and chronological age in a given time period (for instance, 12 months of language growth in 12 months time).

3.1 Results on the Reynell Developmental Language Scales (RDLS)

Studies using the RDLS in deaf children agree that the receptive and expressive language growth (or rate of language development) is roughly half that of peers with normal hearing. Robbins, Svirsky and Kirk (1997), for example, found a receptive language rate of 0.50, meaning about 6 months of growth in 1 year, and an expressive language rate of 0.42, or a growth of about 5 months in 1 year. Before CI children receive their implants, this is their language rate. After implantation, an acceleration of this language development had been reported (Robbins et al. 1997; Miyamoto, Svirsky, & Robbins 1997; Miyamoto, Kirk, Svirsky, & Sehgal 1999; Bollard, Chute, Popp, & Parisier 1999; Robbins, Bollard, & Green 1999; Svirsky, Robbins, Kirk, Pisoni, & Miyamoto 2000a; Kirk, Miyamoto, Lento, Ying, O'Neill, & Fears 2002; Svirsky, Chute, Green, Bollard, & Miyamoto 2000b; Kirk, Miyamoto, Ying, Perdew, & Zuganelis 2000). Rates close to or even greater than those of normally hearing children were found. As a consequence, the gap in absolute scores between children with implants and normally hearing children shown before implantation remained roughly constant after implantation, instead of increasing as in the case of deaf children

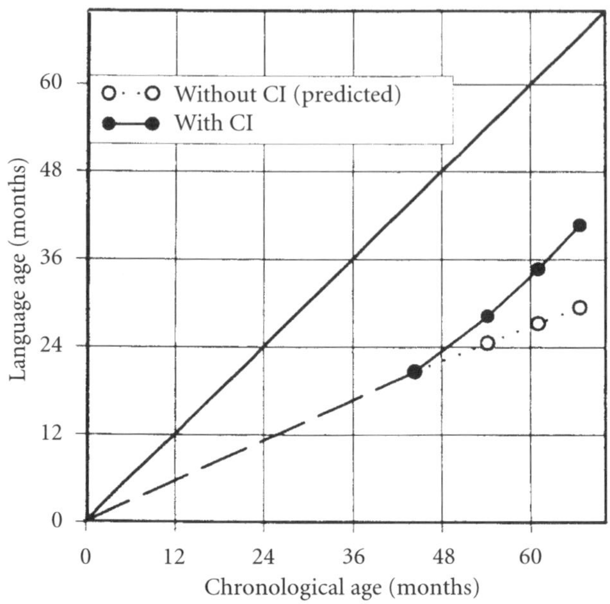

Figure 1. Average language age as a function of chronological age for CI children (black circles). The white circles represent the language growth of deaf children without CI. The solid diagonal line illustrates language growth of normally hearing children (Svirsky et al. 2000a: 156, reprinted with permission from Blackwell Publishing, Oxford).

without implants. Figure 1 (taken from Svirsky et al. 2000a: 156) clearly illustrates these findings. Some studies (Robbins et al. 1999; Svirsky et al. 2000b; Kirk et al. 2002) even indicated that CI children, implanted at approximately 3 years of age, were starting to "catch up" their hearing peers following cochlear implantation, with language rates as high as 1.27 (Svirsky et al. 2000b) and 1.40 (Robbins et al. 1999). These higher-than-normal language rates suggested that the CI children were closing the gap between their language age and their chronological age, a process not completed yet after 4 years of implant use.

3.2 Results on other general language tests

Studies using other tests than the RDLS to assess receptive and/or expressive language in CI children implanted at approximately 4–5 years of age (Geers & Moog 1994; Tomblin, Spencer, Flock, Tyler, & Gantz 1999; Allen & Dyar 1997; Moog & Geers 1999; Moog 2002; Hammes, Novak, Rotz, Willis, Edmondson, &

Thomas 2002; Boothroyd & Boothroyd-Turner 2002) also demonstrated language scores within 2 standard deviations of normally hearing peers (Moog 2002; Moog & Geers 1999) and language learning rates similar to or even greater than those of hearing peers (Hammes et al. 2002) after implantation. The average performance of CI children was at the 70th percentile when compared with profoundly deaf children (Geers & Moog 1994; Boothroyd & Boothroyd-Turner 2002) and at the 2nd percentile when compared with normally hearing children after 3–5 years of implant use.

3.3 Conclusion

These results suggest that early implantation may have a significant impact on language development in children with profound hearing impairment. Since no study to our knowledge has proven that the existing language delay at the moment of implantation can ultimately be reversed, and since only very few studies claim a language rate of more than 1.00, the only way to get rid of the initial delay may well be to prevent it from occurring by very early implantation.

4. Language in CI children: Development in specific sub-domains

4.1 Prelexical babbling

Early vocal development is characterized by the gradual emergence of increasingly complex and speech-like utterances during the first 18 months of life (Oller 1980; Stark 1980). A major landmark in prelexical development is the onset of babbling, which can be defined as the production of adult-like consonant-vowel sequences and typically occurs between 6 and 10 months of age. Babbling utterances are generally recognized as the "foundation" for meaningful words and phonological development: segmental characteristics and syllable shapes found in late prelexical babbling are also common in first words (Vihman, Ferguson, & Elbert 1986). Research in profoundly hearing impaired children has shown that hearing plays a major role in this early vocal development (Oller & Eilers 1988). Indeed, several differences are found in the prelexical utterances of deaf infants compared to normally hearing infants. In general, the early speech of deaf infants is characterized by a late onset of babbling and a low babbling ratio, with reports of delays of as much as 15 to 18 months (Oller & Eilers 1988). Also, the productive output is limited: the size of the consonantal inventory is smaller and hearing impairment alters the nature of place and manner of consonant production (Stoel-Gammon & Otomo 1986). Hearing impaired children have a strong preference for labials over other places of articulation and for nasals over other manners of articulation. Vowels show a tendency towards neutralization, having schwa-like properties. As a consequence, the vowel space is much reduced, with a predominance of mid and central vowels.

It can be anticipated that early cochlear implantation might result in a more normal prelexical vocal development. With regard to onset of babbling, the available studies (Ertmer & Mellon 2001; Ertmer, Young, Grohne, Mellon, Johnson, Corbett, & Saindon 2002; Wright, Purcell, & Reed 2002; Moore & Bass-Ringdahl 2002; Gillis, Schauwers, & Govaerts 2002; Schauwers, Gillis, Daemers, De Beukelaer, & Govaerts 2004) show that only a few months of auditory exposure are needed for CI children to start babbling (ranging on average from 1 to 6.5 months after implantation) regardless of the age at implantation. Consequently, most CI children have a delayed onset of babbling in terms of chronological age, but they start to babble much earlier than normally hearing infants in terms of "hearing age". Moreover, two very early implanted children in the study by Schauwers et al. (2004) who were implanted before the age of 1 year started to babble at a normal chronological age, namely at 8 and 10 months of age. The striking finding that all CI children in these studies started to babble within a short interval of less than 6 months after activation of the implant, irrespective of the age at implantation, is suggestive of a trigger effect of the cochlear implant.

With regard to the segmental characteristics of babbling, children with a CI appeared to babble with greater phonetic diversity than non-implanted hearing impaired infants (Ertmer & Mellon 2001; Ertmer et al. 2002; McCaffrey et al. 1999). Before implantation, the phonetic inventory of CI children was very much like that of profoundly hearing impaired infants. The labial nasal consonant /m/ (SAMPA, www.phon.ucl.ac.uk/home/sampa/home.htm) accounted for 80–90% of all consonants produced and the mid central vowel /@/ accounted for almost 70% of all vowels produced prior to implantation. Relatively soon after activation of the implant however, the strong preference for labials was replaced by a marked increase in "less visible" consonant types like coronals and velars. The large proportion of nasals changed into large proportions of oral stops. Members of the consonant classes that are rare in the babbling of normally hearing infants – fricatives, liquids, and affricates – were also rare in the babbling of CI children. The vowel space expanded from mainly mid central vowels towards a more equal distribution of all vowel categories by the end of the first year of implant use.

Overall, the phonetic inventories of babbling in CI children increase from 2–3 types before implantation to 7–10 types within 1 year after implantation. These increases are in contrast to the decreases in segmental inventories reported for hearing impaired infants (Stoel-Gammon 1988; Stark 1983). Thus, despite the limited number of young CI children studied, the prelexical vocal development of CI infants seems to be significantly different from that of profoundly hearing impaired infants with hearing aids and very similar to the prelexical utterances of normally hearing children.

4.2 Phonological development

A common approach to examine the speech production patterns in children is to investigate the articulatory features (like manner and place of articulation) of vowels and consonants. Three frequently used methods to obtain speech utterances of children in order to examine their segmental characteristics include videotaped spontaneous language samples of unstructured conversations or play situations between the child and a familiar adult (Serry & Blamey 1999; Blamey, Barry, & Jacq 2001; Serry, Blamey, & Grogan 1997; Robinshaw 1996; Grogan, Barker, Dettman, & Blame 1995; Tobey, Geers, & Brenner 1994; Osberger, Robbins, Berry, Todd, Hesketh, & Sedey 1991b; Tobey & Geers 1995; Tye-Murray & Kirk 1993; Tobey & Hasenstab 1991; Geers & Tobey 1992; Tobey, Angelette, Murchison, Nicosia, Sprague, Staller, Brimacombe, & Beiter 1991a), the imitation of CV-syllables (Kirk, Diefendorf, Riley, & Osberger 1995; Sehgal, Kirk, Svirsky, Ertmer, & Osberger 1998; Higgins, Carney, McCleary, & Rogers 1996; Tobey et al. 1994; Tye-Murray, Spencer, Bedia, & Woodworth 1996; Tobey & Geers 1995; Ertmer, Kirk, Sehgal, Riley, & Osberger 1997; Tye-Murray & Kirk 1993; Geers & Tobey 1992; Tobey & Hasenstab 1991; Tobey et al. 1991a), and the elicitation of production of words in isolation by means of picture-naming (Tobey, Pancamo, Staller, Brimacombe, & Beiter 1991b; Chin 2002; Chin 2003; Chin & Kaiser 2000; Kishon-Rabin, Taitelbaum, Muchnik, Gehtler, Kronenberg, & Hildesheimer 2002).

In most studies, the speech samples of the CI children (obtained by means of CV imitations, spontaneous speech recordings, or picture-naming) were analyzed in terms of the percentage of consonant features (manner, place, and voicing) and vowel features (height and place) produced by the child that matched the features of the target. Studies considered bilabial, coronal (or alveolar), palatal, and velar as the possible places of articulation of consonants, and stop, nasal, fricative/affricate, glide, and liquid as the possible manners of articulation of consonants. For example, if the target was /te/ and the child produced /be/, the feature of manner was counted as correct (viz. stop consonant), but no credit was given for the place or voicing feature. With regard to vowels, the place of articulation feature included front, central, and back, and the vowel height feature included high, mid, and low.

A major consequence of deafness in children appears to be a reduced repertoire of sound segments in comparison with normally hearing children. Consonant production in profoundly hearing impaired infants is characterized by a variety of errors, including substitutions of one sound for another, distortions, and omissions of word-final consonants (Osberger & McGarr 1982). Many place-of-articulation errors occur. As in babbling, profoundly hearing impaired infants use visible, front consonants much more frequently than less visible ones, like dorsals (Smith 1975; Gold 1980). Manner-of-articulation errors frequently appear as nasal-oral substitutions. Vowel production in profoundly hearing impaired children is also different from normal speech. A higher proportion of errors is found on vowels requiring a high tongue position than on vowels requiring a central tongue position (Smith 1975). Common processes in the vowel production of hearing impaired children are omissions, tense-lax substitutions, monophthongization of diphthongs and neutralization, which result in the overuse of the vowel /@/.

It was demonstrated earlier that the use of conventional hearing aids was able to improve the production of speech (Geers & Tobey 1992). Cochlear implants, when carefully indicated, give better audiological performance and can be anticipated to contribute even more to a good speech production. Indeed, several studies showed that profoundly hearing impaired children fitted with a CI systematically acquire a diverse set of phonemes involving a wide range of articulatory features. In general, CI children produce 30–40% of consonant features correctly (i.e. matching the target segment) before implantation, and 60–70% after 2–3 years of implant use (Geers & Tobey 1992; Kirk et al. 1995; Sehgal et al. 1998; Chin & Kaiser 2000; Tobey et al. 1994). Scores of over 80% are obtained after 6 years of implant experience (Serry & Blamey 1999; Blamey et al. 2001; Serry et al. 1997). Qualitatively, significant improvements in the percentage of correctly produced consonants are observed for voiceless consonants (mainly voiceless fricatives), less visible coronal consonants (mainly the coronal stops /d/ and /t/), and for all manner categories, but particularly fricatives/affricates, liquids and glides (Geers & Tobey 1992; Sehgal et al. 1998; Tobey et al. 1991b; Chin & Kaiser 2000; Tobey et al. 1994; Osberger et al. 1991b; Tobey & Geers 1995). Vowels are more correctly produced than consonants both before and after implantation. In general, while 30–50% of monophthongs and 20–30% of diphthongs are produced accurately before implantation (Ertmer et al. 1997; Tye-Murray & Kirk 1993; Geers & Tobey 1992), these figures increase to 70–80% and 45–65% respectively after 2–3 years of CI use. Furthermore, evidence exists that these high figures do not even represent plateau levels since Blamey et al. (2001) found accuracies of 92% (monophthongs) and 89% (diphthongs) in CI children who had implant experience of 6 years. In comparison with conventional hearing aid users, CI children display significantly better production of consonant and vowel features than Silver HA users. In fact, the results after 2–3 years of implant use are comparable to those of Gold HA users, with 60–70% correctly produced consonant features and 60–90% correct vowel features (Kirk et al. 1995; Tobey et al. 1994).

Another presentation of phonological development is the construction of a phonetic inventory, in which an inventory is credited with having a consonant or vowel if this segment is produced at least twice, regardless of the target sound ("targetless") or matching the target sound ("target"). Results from such studies of children acquiring English (Serry & Blamey 1999; Blamey et al. 2001; Serry et al. 1997; Chin 2002; Chin 2003) suggest that very few segments are missing from the inventories of CI children implanted at approximately 3.5 years old after 5–6 years of implant use, in contrast to inventories of profoundly hearing impaired infants. Fricatives (/s, z, T, Z/), affricates (/tS/), and the nasal /N/ were lacking the most in most children.

A striking finding by Chin (2002) and Chin (2003) is that some of the CI children produce several non-English sounds, including labiodental stops and fricatives, uvular stops, and palatal and velar fricatives. No good explanation for this could be given.

4.3 Intelligibility

When measuring intelligibility, some CI studies (O'Donoghue, Nikolopoulos, Archbold, & Tait 1999; Allen, Nikolopoulos, & O'Donoghue 2000) rely on judges rating the speech of CI subjects (for instance, the SIR or Speech Intelligibility Rating), but most investigations use identification procedures (also called "write-down" procedures), in which normally hearing listeners are instructed to write down the words or sentences as produced by the child, and in which the intelligibility is indicated by the percentage of (key) words correctly identified (Dawson, Blamey, Dettman, Rowland, Barker, Tobey, Busby, Cowan, & Clark 1995a; Tobey, Geers, Douek, Perrin, Skellett, Brenner, & Toretta 2000; Tobey & Hasenstab 1991; Tobey et al. 1991a; Osberger, et al. 1993; Robbins,

Table 1. An overview of intelligibility scores after 2–3 years of implant use using the McGarr of BIT sentence tests. (Some data regarding younger-implanted CI children are lacking, indicated by a question mark).

	Non-experienced listeners		Experienced listeners	
	Pre-implant	**Post-implant**	**Pre-implant**	**Post-implant**
CI > 5 years	3–7%	15–18% > 4 y CI use: 40%	18%	43%
CI < 5 years	?	48–55% > 4 y CI use: 80%	?	?

Kirk, Osberger & Ertmer 1995; Osberger, Robbins, Todd, & Riley 1994). For the "write-down" method, the available test materials include sentences on the one hand (i.e. the McGarr sentences and the BIT or Beginners' Intelligibility Test) for the subjects to imitate or read, and single words in isolation on the other hand, elicited by imitation or picture-naming. A third possibility is to ask the child to retell a story by means of a set of 4 sequential pictures (i.e. the Story Retell Task), used in the study of Tye-Murray, Spencer and Woodworth (1995). Since many intelligibility assessments make use of adult listeners, it is important to take into account the experience of the listener with speech of children with hearing impairment, as suggested by McGarr (1983) and Monsen (1983).

The variable, that has been found to be highly negatively correlated with speech intelligibility, is degree of hearing loss (Boothroyd 1984; Smith 1975). Profoundly hearing impaired children demonstrate a high level of variation in speech intelligibility: with a consistently found average of merely 20%, with individual scores ranging from 0% to roughly 80% (Smith 1975; Monsen 1978). Typical Gold HA users have 72–81% intelligibility, Silver HA users 20% (Osberger et al. 1993; Osberger et al. 1994; Robbins et al. 1995), and Bronze HA users or typical CI-candidates only 3–7%. After receiving a CI (after the age of 5 years) and using the device for about 2–3 years, the average intelligibility scores increase to 15–18%, a score comparable to that of Silver HA users, but still markedly lower than that of Gold HA users. Cochlear implantation before the age of 5 years, however, resulted in BIT levels comparable to those of Gold HA users (i.e. 80%) after 4–6 years of implant use (Tobey et al. 2000). The overview table (Table 1) also shows that higher intelligibility scores are reported when listeners who are familiar with the speech of children with hearing impairment served as judges (Dawson et al. 1995a).

When using single words as speech material instead of sentences to assess intelligibility (Mondain, Sillon, Vieu, Lanvin, Reuillard-Artieres, Tobey, & Uziel 1997), the findings seem to indicate that children with CI are more intelligible when uttering short sentences than isolated words, similar to normally hearing children.

CI children implanted at an average age of 4.3 years, and tested by means of the intelligibility rating scale SIR (Allen et al. 1998; O'Donoghue et al. 1999) were shown to reach category 2 (unintelligible connected speech with some single words identifiable) one to two years after implantation, category 3 (intelligible connected speech to a listener who concentrated and read lips) 3 to 4 years after CI, and on average category 4 (intelligible speech to a listener with a little experience of deaf speech) five years after implantation.

4.4 Lexical development

Two commonly used vocabulary tests are the *Peabody Picture Vocabulary Test* (PPVT) for receptive vocabulary and the *Expressive One-Word Picture Vocabulary Test* (EOWPVT) for expressive vocabulary. Similar to the general language test RDLS (described in Section 3.1), the raw scores on these tests are converted to age-equivalent scores based on normative tables for normally hearing subjects and to vocabulary rates.

Several studies (Boothroyd, Geers, & Moog 1991; Dawson, Blamey, Dettman, Barker, & Clark 1995b; Geers & Moog 1994) have documented that the rate of lexical development of deaf children was only a fraction of the average rate in normally hearing children, viz. 0.33–0.63. Hence, CI candidates have a substantial vocabulary delay before implantation, but after implantation they have been shown to develop vocabulary skills significantly faster than their peers without implants (Kuo & Gibson 2000; Dawson et al. 1995b; El-Hakim, Levasseur, Papsin, Panesar, Mount, Stevens, & Harrison 2001; Geers & Moog 1994). Receptive and expressive vocabulary rates between 0.71 and 1.1 were found for CI children implanted between 3 and 9 years of age, a pace not significantly different from normally hearing children.

Sometimes, even higher than normal rates were found (Bollard, Chute, Popp, & Parisier 1999; Kuo & Gibson 2000; Kirk et al. 2000). In the study of Bollard et al. (1999), for instance, the children showed a mean vocabulary age of 12.4 months before implantation (at a chronological age of 36 months). At the end of 18 months of implant use, they reached a mean vocabulary age of 55 months and had equaled their hearing peers in vocabulary acquisition. Thus, the initial gap between chronological age and vocabulary age before implantation did not increase (and even decreased) after children started using the device, as it would have if they had not received CI at all.

Another measure on the lexical level is the type/token ratio (TTR), used in the studies of Szagun (2000) (studying German-learning children) and Ertmer, Strong and Sadagopan (2003). This is a measure of vocabulary diversity based on the ratio of different words (types) to the total number of words (tokens) in a sample. We have to take into account, however, that the TTR is function of the number of tokens in the language sample: samples containing larger numbers of tokens give lower values for TTR and vice versa. Although the TTR's of CI children were quite similar to the ratios for normally hearing children when considering hearing age (i.e. number of months after implantation), the TTR's were based on far fewer word types and tokens per sample than normally hearing children. For instance, normally hearing German-learning children had a vocabulary of approximately 400 word tokens at 29.5 months of age, in contrast to approximately 250 word tokens for the CI group at 18.5 months after implantation (or at 30 months chronological age) (Szagun 2001). In addition, a number of studies (Coerts, Baker, van den Broek, & Brokx 1996; Szagun 2000) agreed that CI children had a marked preference for content words over function words both before and after implantation. This could be a result of their impaired hearing, as content words can receive stress and are therefore perceptually more salient than function words, which are normally unstressed.

4.5 Morphosyntactic development

Mean Length of Utterance (MLU) measured in morphemes is commonly used as a general indicator of grammatical progress. In a number of studies (Szagun 1997; Szagun 2000; Szagun 2001; Coerts et al. 1996; Ertmer et al. 2003; Spencer, Tye-Murray, & Tomblin 1998; Coerts & Mills 1994), MLU was calculated on spontaneous speech samples of CI children. Although every study demonstrated an increase in MLU after implantation, the results across studies showed great diversity, and among CI children the variability was large: some CI children progressed as rapidly as normally hearing children, others were much slower in their morphologic and syntactic development. Table 2 demonstrates these substantial differences in MLU results across studies.

Although it is difficult to compare MLU over different languages, all investigators agree that CI children make progress in combining morphemes, but the intersubject variability appears to be very large. In addition, the data show that CI children acquire the morphosyntax of their language more slowly than normally hearing children with a considerable delay in MLU in compar-

Table 2. Overview of MLU results in CI children acquiring English (E), German (G) or Dutch (D).

Mean age at implantation	Number of months after CI	Mean MLU	Study
1;8	42	2.57	Ertmer et al. 2003 (E)
2;3	18	≤ 1.50–3.25	Szagun 2000 (G)
2;6	24	4.30	Szagun 1997 (G)
2;5	32	3.50	Szagun 2001 (G)
3;1	18	4.80 (in words)	Bollard et al. 1999 (E)
3;4	42	2.70	Szagun 1997 (G)
5;0	18	1.69–1.87	Coerts et al. 1996 (D)
5;4	18	> 4.00	Coerts & Mills 1994 (D)
5;7	46	2.55–8.96	Spencer et al. 1998 (E)

ison with normally hearing children. Many CI children (implanted at a mean age of 2.4 years) remain at the stage of two-word utterances (i.e. MLU of ≤ 2.25) after several years of implant use, while most normally hearing children reach the stage of complex grammar (i.e. MLU of > 4.00) by the age of 3 years (Szagun 2001).

The MLU is a rather general and quantitative measure, and more detailed qualitative analysis of the morphosyntactic development in CI children can be done (Coerts et al. 1996; Szagun 2000; Szagun 1997; Spencer et al. 1998; Svirsky, Stallings, Lento, Ying, & Leonard 2002). Such studies have shown that English-learning CI children acquire plural formation on nouns earlier and more easily than the regular past tense marker on main verbs (Svirsky et al. 2002; Spencer et al. 1998), similar to normally hearing children. With respect to case and gender marking in German (Szagun 2000), most CI children acquire the nominative case of the definite (/der/, /die/, /das/) and indefinite (/ein/, /eine/, /ein/) articles. However, accusative forms are rare and dative forms absent. Additionally, the CI children acquire more definite forms when these are used in pronominal function than in article function.

The above-mentioned studies explain the morphological acquisition order by the degree of perceptual salience of the grammatical cues. For example, regular past tense in English is marked by the addition of a final /t/ or /d/, both characterized by a brief burst and formant transition lasting a few tens of milliseconds. In contrast, the noun plurals are marked by the addition of a final /s/ or /z/. These phonemes have a much longer duration than the bursts associated with a final /t/ or /d/. Therefore, Svirsky et al. (2002) assumed that the morphological marker for plurals was perceptually more prominent to the CI users than the marker for past tense. Similarly, Szagun (2000) predicted that CI children would have problems acquiring inflectional morphemes on unstressed function words, such as articles. German case inflection, for instance, occurs mainly on articles, so she expected CI children to have particular problems in acquiring case inflection, which was confirmed by the results. The CI children perform nearly as well as normally hearing children in acquiring noun plurals and verb inflectional morphology on the main verb (viz. infinitive /en/, third person singular, imperative singular, past particle, first person singular, in this order). However, they acquire substantially less forms of the definite and indefinite articles, particularly case-inflected forms, since articles do not receive stress. The fact that the children acquire more forms of the definite article when used pronominally is an additional evidence for the effect of perceptual salience.

These suggestions made by Svirsky et al. (2002) and Szagun (2000) call for cross-linguistic research to investigate the possible universality of the factor of perceptual prominence in the development of grammar.

4.6 Pragmatic development

4.6.1 *Communicative behaviors*

Important features of (preverbal) interaction in children include the ability to distribute attention between the parent and objects of communication (which occurs at around 4 to 6 months of age in normally hearing children, when the child begins to follow the parent's line of gaze), the ability of turn-taking by gesture and by vocalization, and the awareness of the appropriate time to take a turn (Bruner 1983).

Methods to quantify these features in young children have been developed by Tait and colleagues (Tait 1993; Tait & Lutman 1994; Lutman & Tait 1995; Tait, Lutman, & Robinson 2000). Transcribed recordings of conversations are scored according to a detailed written protocol. The turns taken are identified and classified as vocal (VTT or vocal turn taking) or gestural (GTT) according to whether they are taken using voice or silent gesture or sign. If turns contain elements that cannot be predicted from the adult's preceding turn, they are further classified as showing autonomy (vocal VA, or gestural GA), including contradicting the adult, introducing new topics or information, joking, or asking questions. A child who is not yet using words can nevertheless exercise vocal autonomy, for example by vocalizing strongly to attract attention. When a turn is taken vocally without simultaneous eye contact between the child and the adult, it is classified as a non-looking turn (NLT). Finally, the percentage of

A: You went to tea with Susie, didn't you! ↓

C: Linda house, Linda.

A: Wasn't Linda there? ↓ Wasn't she? Was Pamela

C: (shakes head)

A: there? ↓ I know, you're Susie's friend. Was

C: I Susie friend.

A: Pamela there? ↓

C: Pamela school.

Figure 2. Transcript of a conversational interaction between adult (A) and child (C). Arrows indicate turn-taking by the child, dotted and solid lines indicate eye contact (see text). The arrows mark 4 occasions when the child takes a conversational turn: 3 of these turns are vocal and 1 gestural (shown in brackets); the first turn is a non-looking turn; 3 of the 4 turns show autonomy, by introducing new information (adopted from Tait 1993).

the total number of adult's syllables for which the child is looking at the adult is calculated (eye contact or EC).

Figure 2 illustrates the scoring. The transcript shows the adult's (A) and the child's (C) contributions presented in parallel. Arrows (↓) mark the child's opportunity for a conversational turn. The eye contact is added to the transcript as a dotted line just under the adult's words (or part of words) for which the child is looking at the adult, and as a continuous line under the words for which the child is not looking at the adult.

This type of analysis has shown that three measures (VTT, VA, and NLT) increase substantially within the first year after implantation in children implanted at a mean age of 3.3 years (Tait 1993; Tait & Lutman 1994). Vocal turns increase to 80–90% of all turns taken at 6–12 months post CI, and autonomy and non-looking turns reach approximately 50% of all turns taken at 3–6 months post CI. This is very similar to the results of Gold/Silver hearing aid users: both groups show increased ability to contribute vocally in conversation, and to make these vocalizations even without looking at the adult speaker. Bronze hearing aid users in contrast, do not develop this ability: they show a substantial increase in GTT and GA. These latter measures decrease for the

CI group. In other words, CI candidates resemble Bronze hearing aid users in their preference for gestural modes of communication, but after implantation, they rapidly move towards the vocal and auditory modes as seen in the Silver and Gold group and they may even exceed them. The remaining measure, EC, tends to increase slightly for all groups, but this appears to be a very idiosyncratic measure with very large variation. As a group, the CI children have a lower level of EC, relative to the Gold/Silver HA group, which may indicate that watching the speaker is less important for implantees.

4.6.2 *Narratives*

A narrative can be defined as a discourse form in which at least two different events are described so that the relationship between them (temporal, causal, contrastive) becomes clear. It is expected to contain an introduction and an organized sequence of events that leads to a logical conclusion. The development of narrative skills relies largely on incidental learning, resulting from repeated exposure to a number of different types of story forms. Deaf children are reported to have difficulties in developing the narrative structures, clearly because of their limited access to verbal information and thus to incidental learning (Yoshinaga-Itano & Snyder 1985; Griffith, Ripich, & Dastoli 1990; King & Quigley 1985; Marschark, Mouradian, & Halas 1994; Klecan-Aker & Blondeau 1990). In consequence, they produce fewer propositions, shorter or incomplete sentences with less structural variability, they omit adverbs and conjunctions, and have difficulty with evaluative elements. The narrative ability in 8-to-9-year-old CI children (implanted at a mean age of 3,5 years) was assessed by asking them to tell a story after viewing an eight-picture sequence story (Crosson & Geers 2000 and Crosson & Geers 2001). Each utterance was coded for type of narrative structure: (1) *orientations* (which provide the setting of the narrative), (2) *complicating actions* (which refer to a chronologically ordered event), (3) *evaluations* (which provide the characters' reactions to events), or (4) *resolutions* (which occur after the high point, resolving the action). In addition, the use of conjunctions and referents (such as nominals, pronouns, modifiers) was analyzed as measure of cohesion. The results showed a correlation between the narrative ability of the CI children after 4 to 6 years of implant use with the speech perception. Children with more auditory benefit from their cochlear implant use fewer orientations (30% in comparison with 46% in "poor perceivers"), more evaluations (28% in comparison with 19% in "poor perceivers"), and are more likely to recruit both coordinating and temporal conjunctions to link semantic relations in their narratives. Thus, these "good perceivers" structure their stories in a more normal pattern (i.e.

22% orientations and 30% evaluations) than below-average speech perceivers. And although their use of subordinate conjunctions may be not as well developed as in hearing children, it is significantly above that of deaf children with below-average auditory benefit of their implant. In addition is shown that good narrative ability adds to reading comprehension scores, supporting the importance of narrative skills to academic achievement.

5. Factors affecting language outcomes in CI children

One the most consistent findings reported in studies on pediatric CI is the large variability and individual differences in outcome performance observed on a wide range of language measures. Some children do very well with their implants, and other children do poorly. At present, a good understanding or explanation for these large individual differences does not exist, but several factors have already been identified that are responsible for the variation in performance, and will be described in this section.

5.1 Age at implantation

Evidence exists that children who receive a CI at a younger age do better on a range of language measures than children who are implanted at an older age. In general, early implantation increases the likelihood to obtain age-appropriate language skills.

With regard to the onset of babbling, Schauwers et al. (2004) showed that it takes a median of 1 month of auditory exposure to start babbling, regardless of the age at implantation. However, since babbling in normally hearing children starts at a mean age of 8 months, early cochlear implantation is mandatory to have the child babbling at a normal age. This was the case for the two youngest CI subjects (implanted at 5 and 7 months of age), who started babbling at 8 and 10 months of age, and who thus took their first steps to a normal speech and language development at a normal chronological age.

Only few studies addressed other linguistic domains as a function of age at implantation, and the findings are not unequivocal. But it has to be noted that most reports focused on children who were implanted late in terms of linguistic development. Implantation beyond the age of 2 or 4 years may be too late for a number of speech developmental features. Some investigators found more improvements in segmental speech aspects in the younger CI groups (i.e. implanted before 5–9! years of age) (Kirk & Hill-Brown 1985; Tobey et al. 1991a;

Tye-Murray et al. 1995; Grogan et al. 1995; Tobey et al. 1991b), while others (Blamey et al. 2001) found no evidence of significant differences in the production of vowels and consonants in a group of CI children implanted between 2 and 5 years of age.

With regard to intelligibility scores using the McGarr or BIT sentence tests, implantation before the age of 5 years yields 48–55% scores, compared to 15–18% when implanted after 5 years of age (Dawson et al. 1995a; Osberger et al. 1994)! The intelligibility also seems to improve faster when implanted at a young age (before 5 years) (Tye-Murray et al. 1995), as do the receptive and expressive language measures (by means of the RDLS) (Kirk et al. 2000; Kirk et al. 2002; Hammes et al. 2002; Kuo & Gibson 2000). On the other hand, no such age benefit was found for vocabulary growth (Miyamoto et al. 1999; El-Hakim et al. 2001; Dawson et al. 1995b) and only a weak benefit for the measure MLU (Szagun 2001). With regard to communicative behavior, autonomous vocal or gestural turn-takings are significantly higher in earlier-implanted children (in the range of 2–5 years) (Tait et al. 2000).

Two interesting factors have been postulated to contribute to this alleged age benefit. First, cochlear implantation at very young ages facilitates the natural ability of young children to learn incidentally, an ability that decreases with age. Older children depend more on didactic instruction and it has been shown that this method is less effective for true language mastery than incidental learning (Robbins et al. 1999). Secondly, early auditory stimulation through a CI contributes to more normal maturation of the auditory pathways. Electrophysiological measures (of the auditory cortex) have suggested a maturational delay in implanted children that approximates the period of auditory deprivation prior to implantation (Robinson 1998). As a consequence, this maturational delay will be smaller in children implanted at younger ages.

5.2 Educational approaches

Geers (2002) and Geers, Brenner, Nicholas, Uchanski, Tye-Murray and Tobey (2002) performed a large-scale study to investigate factors contributing to auditory, speech, language, and reading outcomes after 4 to 6 years of CI use in 136 children with prelingual deafness (all aged 8–9 years at the time of testing). The careful analysis focused on the identification of the educational factors most conducive to maximum implant benefit. It turned out that the educational variables accounted for approximately 12% of the variance in outcome after implantation. The primary rehabilitative factor associated with performance outcome was educational emphasis on oral communication (OC). This was more important than any other rehabilitative factor examined, including classroom placement (public or private, special education or mainstream), amount of therapy, experience of the therapist, and parent participation in therapy. This is in line with other studies that have shown that implanted children who were immersed in OC environments tend to develop much better expressive language (in terms of vocabulary, segmental content and intelligibility) than implanted children who were placed in total communication (TC) programs (which imply the integration of spoken and signed language) (Robbins et al. 1997; Miyamoto et al. 1999; Robbins et al. 1999; Svirsky et al. 2000a; Kirk et al. 2002; Cullington, Hodges, Butts, Dolan-Ash, & Balkany 2000; Osberger et al. 1994; Tobey et al. 2000; Osberger et al. 1993; Chin 2002 and Chin 2003). On the other hand, receptive language skills are not significantly different for OC and TC children (Cullington et al. 2000; Dawson et al. 1995b).

An obvious explanation for the discrepancy in expressive language abilities between OC and TC children could relate to the nature and extent of the language to which the children are exposed. Whereas oral children with hearing parents are exposed to spoken communication throughout the day, it is often the case that children who use TC have a more limited exposure to language. Many caregivers of children who use total communication are learning signed language at the same time as their child, thus offering an impoverished model to the child. Furthermore, it is often the case that only a limited number of people in the child's environment know or are learning signs. It may be that the linguistic environment of many children who use TC is impoverished in comparison to that of OC children and of normally hearing peers. However, this issue needs further study.

5.3 Implant characteristics

Approximately 24% of the variance in outcome of implantation (speech perception, speech production, spoken language, simultaneous language, and reading) can be predicted by device-specific features (Geers 2002 and Geers et al. 2002) such as coding strategies, the number of active electrodes, the extent of the dynamic range and loudness growth.

5.4 Child characteristics

The most important child-related predictor of cochlear implant outcome seems to be good nonverbal intelligence (Geers 2002; Geers et al. 2002). Once this variable was held constant, other features like age at implantation and age at onset of deafness did not contribute significantly to speech perception and speech production skill levels measured at ages 8–9 after 5.5 years of implant use! Family-related features like family size and parent's education did not seem to provide a particular (dis)advantage. All child and family characteristics together (and thus primarily IQ) accounted for 18% of the outcome variance after implantation in this study.

5.5 Level of pre-operative hearing

Children with more residual hearing prior to implantation show better achievements than children with less residual hearing. Szagun (2001) found that pre-operative hearing correlates significantly with linguistic growth in MLU (assessed by means of spontaneous language samples) and with vocabulary growth (assessed by parental report), accounting for 53% and 42% of the variability respectively. In other words, better pre-operative hearing is associated with more rapid growth in grammar and vocabulary. These correlations are much stronger than the ones for age at implantation (for children implanted between 14–46 months). Similarly, El-Hakim et al. (2001) demonstrated that residual hearing is the only significant predictive factor for expressive vocabulary performance on the EOWPVT test for children implanted at approximately 5 years of age.

5.6 Length of CI experience

Longitudinal studies of CI children (Tomblin et al. 1999) reported that length of implant use, rather than chronological age, is the principal factor accounting for the variance in the performance on syntactic tests of children with cochlear implants. That is, deaf children with CI experience have better English grammar than those without CI experience and the more CI experience the better the grammar. The use of morphological inflected endings, studied by Spencer et al. (1998), is not related to the age of the CI children, but to the length of CI experience. The investigators particularly found significant correlations between CI experience and use of third person singular tense and total bound morphemes used. These findings suggest that use of English inflected endings may be less affected by maturation and aging, and more by auditory input.

5.7 Speech perception

Children with better speech perception tend to include more English inflected endings within conversation (Spencer et al. 1998). Furthermore, open-set speech perception scores, as assessed by Moog and Geers (1999), correlate significantly with scores on measures of speech production, language, and reading. With regard to narratives, Crosson and Geers (2001) revealed a significant difference between good speech perceivers and poor speech perceivers in narrative structure and cohesion. The narrative structure of the good perceivers is similar to that of normally hearing children and different from that of poor perceivers, in that it includes less orientations (which provide the setting of the narrative) and more evaluations (which provide the characters' reactions to events). The CI children with better speech perception also use more conjunctions and more referents, which are both signs of cohesion in a narrative.

5.8 Higher-level cognitive factors

Pisoni, Cleary, Geers and Tobey (1999) believe that individual variation in performance of CI children be related to processing information at more central levels of analysis that reflect the operation of cognitive processes such as perception, attention, learning, and memory. They criticize studies that focus on demographic variables and traditional outcome measures, because these measures of performance are argued to be the final "product" of a large number of complex sensory, perceptual, cognitive processes that may be responsible for the observed variation among CI users. Instead, Pisoni et al. (1999) prefer to focus on "processes" that lead to a final response, on the underlying mechanisms used to perceive and produce spoken language. A series of correlational analyses on test scores (of speech perception, language comprehension, spoken word recognition, receptive vocabulary, receptive and expressive language development, and speech intelligibility) in "Star" CI children (i.e. who scored in the upper 20% on an open-set speech perception test), and "Controls" (i.e. who scored in the lower 20% on an open-set speech perception test) suggested that the exceptionally good performance of the "Stars" might be due to their superior abilities to process spoken language, specifically, to perceive, encode, and retrieve phonological representations of spoken words from lexical memory and use these representations in a variety of different language processing tasks, especially tasks that depend on vocal learning and phonological processing. Secondly, Pisoni et al. (1999) reported correlations between measures of working memory, in which digit span was assessed, and four sets of outcome measures, namely speech perception, speech production, language, and reading. Moderate to high correlations were found between forward auditory digit span and each of the 4 outcome measures. This suggests the presence of a common source of variance related to working memory, viz. the encoding and rehearsal of phonological representations of spoken words. The performance differences among CI children can be due to the operation of a subcomponent of working memory known as the "phonological loop", which is responsible for the rehearsal and maintenance of the phonological representations of spoken words in memory. The authors also suggest that rehearsal speed in working memory may be one of the factors that distinguished good CI users from poorer ones. The additional correlation between digit span and communication mode suggests that early auditory experience in oral-only programs may have specific effects on working memory capacity: OC children have significantly longer digit spans than TC children. With these findings, Pisoni et al. (1999) want to emphasize that traditional outcome measures are not adequate to assess these underlying processes and may be unable to detect and measure important central cognitive factors as sources of variance.

6. Conclusion

Cochlear implantation is a major event in the life of a deaf-born child and it is likely to have a significant impact on his/her further development. Although impressive amounts of data have been reported to date, the interpretation remains difficult. This is mainly due to the fact that almost every element in this field is in full evolution, jeopardizing the comparability of data. The technology of implantation has gone through important steps of amelioration, our insights in the early speech and language development have evolved substantially, universal neonatal screening programs have realized early detection of hearing impairment, early intervention has become possible and the indications for cochlear implantation have extended towards low ages. On top of that, we are dealing with children in full development and it is difficult to know for sure whether an evolution in such a child is to be attributed to the intervention or to the natural development.

Notwithstanding these difficulties, the available data show clear evidence of the significant impact of cochlear implantation on the speech and language development of the child. Congenitally deaf children develop delays in almost all aspects of their linguistic evolution. After implantation, the rate of development tends to normalize. This is demonstrated by overall measures of the receptive and productive speech development and also by more specific linguistic measures. The phonology shows a significant increase in the percentage of correct consonant and vowel production and an increase to a near to normal phonetic inventory. The intelligibility of the child's words increases, as does his or her lexical development. Also the morphosyntax benefits from implantation, although this issue seems to remain difficult and most implanted children seem to dwell at the stage of 2-word utterances for a long time. This also seems to be the case for the pragmatic development, where benefits are seen but they seem to be subject to ceiling effects. Ceiling effects are very important and to date, it is insufficiently clear to which extend they exist in this domain. Indeed, cochlear implantation may speed up the development to near to normal rates, but a crucial question remains whether the delays, as they have been built up prior to implantation, are reversible and will disappear. So far, in most aspects of the linguistic development, this seems NOT to be the case. On the other hand, it cannot be overemphasized that almost all available data are from children who received their implant between 2 and 5 years of age, ages that can be considered late in terms of linguistic development. One could anticipate by extrapolation that earlier implantation would imply smaller delays to start with, and thus better outcomes. Age at implantation has been shown to be a significant predictive factor, but not the only one. The outcome also depends to a great extend on technological features (like speech coding strategies), on the educational setting and on the cognitive skills of the child.

Above all, and probably the quintessence of the whole issue, is the awareness that the developmental path of a child, not only in linguistic terms, depends largely on the natural ability of a child to learn incidentally rather than by didactic instruction, as mentioned by Robbins et al. (1999). From a developmental point of view, the linguistic acquisitions of a deaf child may teach us how far we can get with didactic instruction, and what its limit is. Cochlear implants, by restoring hearing, may restore the facility of incidental learning and the earlier this is done, the better it may be for the child.

Critical periods in the acquisition of lexical skills

Evidence from deaf individuals

Amy R. Lederberg and Patricia E. Spencer

1. Introduction

The speed with which young children acquire language is one of the most remarkable feats of early childhood. Is this ability unique to early childhood? Lenneberg (1967) initiated the recent surge of interest in the hypothesis that the ability to acquire language is time limited. Based on language acquisition research with children with brain injuries, those with Down syndrome, and those that become deafened during development, he suggested that exposure to linguistic input has to occur before the age of 12 years in order to reach native proficiency. He posited that the brain plasticity necessary for language development declines precipitously with puberty. This so-called "critical period" hypothesis is thought to be applicable to acquisition of both first and second languages. With hearing children, except for children who have cognitive impairments like the ones studied by Lenneberg, and case studies of children isolated from language because of child abuse (e.g., Genie as described in Curtiss 1977), researchers have studied this hypothesis by focusing primarily on second language learning. In contrast, deaf children provide unique opportunities to address issues about the critical period hypothesis as it relates to learning a first language.

Since Lenneberg's (1967) original formulation, empirical and theoretical work has refined the definition of a critical period (Bailey, Bruer, Symons, & Lichtman 2001; Newport, Bavelier, & Neville 2001). Rather than a period that is characterized by an abrupt end to learning ability, the ability to learn from environmental input is seen as declining more gradually. For example, Newport et al. (2001) defined a critical period as "a peak period of plasticity, occur-

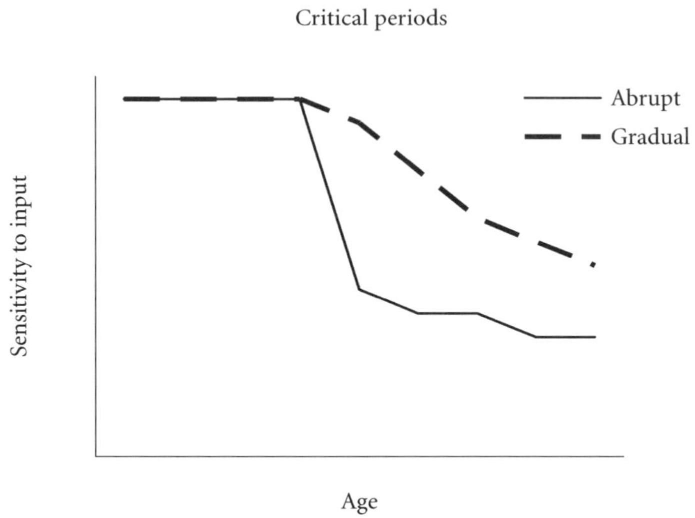

Figure 1. Different shapes of possible critical periods

ring at some maturationally defined time in development, followed by reduced plasticity later in life" (p. 482). A critical period is indicated when there is a heightened sensitivity to environmental input during a specific time period in development followed by a substantial decrease in the ability to learn from that input. Although in some cases this decrease happens abruptly at a specific age, the decline in plasticity can also occur gradually over long periods of time (see Figure 1).

Experimental evidence for critical periods should show that "the same experience at different stages of development results in significant long-term differences in performance, behavior, or brain structure" (Bruer 2001:24). It is not necessary to show that learning is impossible after the critical period; rather that learning occurs more rapidly and with increased organization if it occurs at the time of heightened sensitivity. Although some researchers and clinicians distinguish between "sensitive" and "critical" periods based on the degree to which learning can occur outside a specified time period, current thinking about the phenomenon make such a distinction more apparent than real (Newport et al. 2001). Therefore, the term "critical period" will be used throughout this paper.

It is important to keep in mind that evidence for critical periods does not have implications for the underlying acquisition process (Bailey et al. 2001; Newport et al. 2001). Although Lenneberg (1967) proposed that linguistic critical periods were due to maturational changes in the brain's plasticity, others have shown that critical periods could equally result from changes in plasticity due to early learning (Seidenberg 2003, April). As neural structures and functions begin to specialize based on early experience, it may become increasingly arduous for a re-organization to occur.

Research on language of deaf people is uniquely well-suited to the study of critical periods because of the variation within that group in their initial exposure to language in a form that they are able to receive and process. Deaf children with deaf parents are typically exposed to sign language from the time of birth and their language development is remarkably similar to hearing children's development of spoken language (Emmorey 2002; Meadow-Orlans, Spencer, & Koester in press). On the other hand, more than ninety percent of deaf children have hearing parents and experience delays in their exposure to language input because they cannot perceive the spoken language in their environment (Spencer & Lederberg 1997). For these children, exposure to language occurs only after their hearing loss is identified and they are placed in an intervention environment that provides accessible language. This can happen anytime from infancy through adulthood.

Defining the nature of language input for deaf children can be difficult. Traditional amplification (hearing aids) and even use of cochlear implants typically fails to provide deaf children with the same complete and finely differentiated auditory language input that occurs effortlessly for hearing children (see Schauwers, Gillis, & Govaerts this volume). Therefore, deaf children with hearing parents almost always receive, at best, an incomplete and auditorily distorted model of spoken language. Even when their hearing parents learn sign language, the language environment of deaf children with hearing parents is rarely as rich as that provided to most hearing children. When hearing parents are new learners of sign, they tend to be non-fluent and to therefore present a less than complete representation of the intended language (Lederberg & Everhart 1998; Spencer 1993; Swisher & Christie 1989). Deaf children in environments with fluently signing deaf teachers and peers rarely experience the same type of interactive linguistic input that deaf children receive from their deaf parents. Therefore, in considering the concept of a critical period, the nature of linguistic input must be considered. The fact that deaf children of hearing parents as a group tend to fail to attain native competency (evidenced by language levels that are lower than that of deaf children of deaf parents or of hearing children) is not necessarily evidence of a critical period, because the input may not provide a complete language model. Rather, a critical period is indicated when different rates of development and different levels of competency are observed among deaf children who have similar language exposures but differ on age of initial exposure.

2. Critical periods and semantic abilities

Research on the effects of age of exposure on deaf children's language development has almost exclusively focused on grammatical skills, with evidence suggesting that late exposure to language affects the ultimate mastery of grammatical systems in sign language (Emmorey, Bellugi, Friederici, & Horn 1995; Mayberry & Lock 2003; Morford 2003; Newport 1990). In fact, in their review on critical periods in deaf individuals, Newport et al. (2001) concluded, in contrast to grammatical competence, "the acquisition of vocabulary and semantic processing occur relatively normally in late learners" (p. 484). Indeed, we agree that lexical knowledge relative to grammatical knowledge is resilient to variations in age of exposure. However, this does not mean lexical skills are unaffected by late exposure to language. Reports of deaf children's vocabulary development show a rate of acquisition of words to be generally 40 to 60 percent of that of hearing children, even when the children are provided with consistent amplification and high quality programming (Blamey 2003; Geers & Moog 1994; Lederberg & Spencer 2001; Moeller, Osberger, & Eccarius 1986). Problems with vocabulary learning are assumed to be a result of environmental factors (e.g., less exposure to words in the environment because of poor input or hearing loss, poor reading abilities). However, there also may be fundamental problems with vocabulary learning due to critical period effects.

What does it mean to say there is a critical period for vocabulary? In her argument against such a notion, Fischer (1998) points out that the ability to acquire new vocabulary does not disappear or even decrease with development. Throughout the lifespan, adults acquire new words and assign new meanings to old words. However, the issue explored here is whether that ability is the same no matter when an individual is initially exposed to and starts to learn a first language. Vocabulary mastery or semantic competence is also multi-faceted, with the possibility that only some aspects are sensitive to the timing of first language acquisition. Evidence for a critical period would include age of exposure effects on adult lexical knowledge or lexicon size, on the growth rate of lexical acquisition, on the ability to process the meaning of words and on word learning processes available to learn new words.

Quasi-experimental evidence for critical periods can result from investigations of associations between deaf people's language competence and the age they were exposed to their first language (Newport 1991). Deaf children gain access to linguistic input in three ways: (1) by being integrated into a community that uses a sign language to communicate (2) by being identified as having a hearing loss and gaining access to language through appropriate intervention services including use of hearing aids and/or sign (3) by receiving a cochlear implant that increases access to spoken language. The effect of age of exposure on lexical skills can be explored within each of these ways deaf people gain access to a first language.

2.1 Evidence from sign language

Historically, most deaf children with profound or severe-profound hearing losses were first raised in an "oral only" environment, but amplification typically failed to provide sufficient input for understanding spoken language. For many, exposure to accessible language did not occur until they left their family of origin and gained access to the deaf community (usually in residential schools) and were exposed to sign language (Mayberry & Fischer 1989). Thus, among the current generation of older deaf adults, age at which they were exposed to accessible language varied from birth (for those with deaf parents) through adulthood. Deaf adults who had hearing parents typically spent extended periods of time in language-deprived environments. An exploration of the skills deaf individuals develop while language deprived will illuminate what they bring to the language learning task when they finally are exposed to language, and thus provide a context for understanding the effect of age of exposure on language acquisition.

2.1.1 *Gestural systems prior to linguistic exposure*

Deaf children who are deprived of accessible linguistic input still communicated with others in their environment (Goldin-Meadow 2003). At the time of language exposure, these non-linguistic communication systems served as the foundation for language development. Both hearing and deaf children begin communication by gesturing, but for typically developing children, gestures become supportive of linguistic (spoken or sign) development (Capone & McGregor 2004). For language-deprived deaf children, the simple gestures of infancy frequently develop into a more complex gestural communication system, referred to as "homesigns" by the deaf community. Examples of these idiosyncratic gestural systems have been observed in many countries around the world (Morford 1996). Research on homesigns has primarily focused on the structure (similar to grammatical properties) of these systems. However, the nature of the nonlinguistic "lexicon" of these systems can be inferred from these reports.

Goldin-Meadow and her colleagues have analyzed in detail the homesigns of four American preschoolers without access to spoken or sign language (Goldin-Meadow 2003; Goldin-Meadow, Mylander, & Butcher 1995; Morford & Goldin-Meadow 1997). During free play, the children used points most frequently for communication, typically to refer to entities that are nouns in language, as well as spatial locations. They occasionally used points to represent nonpresent entities (e.g., pointing to a pig's head to refer to a hat that is typically on the pig). In addition, on average, the children used 25 iconic representational gestures per one- to two-hour observation. About 25% of these gestures were American conventional gestures and were stable in both form and meaning. Conventional gestures were used to represent both the conventional meaning (e.g., holding finger up to mean "wait") and related, but broader meanings (e.g., "wait" for future tense, such as gesturing "wait" to indicate the child was about to go to a bag to get something (Goldin-Meadow 2003: 80). Finally, the children used iconic, structured, pantomimic gestures that depicted actions and perceptual attributes of referents (e.g., twisting hand motion to indicate opening a jar). These gestures were not like the free-formed pantomime that hearing individuals produce when communicating solely through gestures (e.g., charades). Rather the homesigns were a combination of a restricted set of handshapes and actions. These sublexical components had predictable meanings that corresponded with a class of referents (e.g., a fist indicated handling an object that was skinny and long), and thus resembled classifiers in sign languages (Emmorey 2002). Homesign systems allowed the deaf children to express a range of semantic intentions with a limited lexicon.

Case studies of deaf adolescents and adults in other countries suggest that older deaf people who have family members willing to use homesign develop an even more elaborate homesign system (Morford 1996). Homesign lexicons are still much smaller and less explicit compared to language or even the gestures of hearing people who know a language but are instructed to communicate solely through gestures (Morford, Singleton, & Goldin-Meadow 1995b). Nevertheless, homesigners bring to the language learning task a representational system that may facilitate the acquisition of linguistic lexical items at the age of exposure. In fact, Goldin-Meadow (2003) and Morford (2003) argue that the homesigners have foundational representational skills and do not enter the language-learning task at the level of nonverbal hearing toddlers. For instance, homesigners understand that conventional symbols are used to refer to categories of referents and that the same symbol (like the gesture for "wait") can have more than one meaning. In addition, homesigns have a language-like morphological structure. On the other hand, unlike linguistic signs, homesigns may lack a purely formal (non-meaning based) phonological sublexical structure (Mayberry 2002; Morford 1996).

Longitudinal research with one of the four American preschoolers studied by Goldin-Meadow (2003) suggests that homesign can be used to facilitate acquisition of a formal linguistic system. This child, known as David, was reassessed at 9.5 years when he had only had minimal contact with ASL and then again when he was 23 years old (Morford, Singleton, & Goldin-Meadow 1995a). David had had some, limited, exposure to sign in high school and then attended a college program for deaf students from 18 to 23 years old, and thus was immersed in ASL as an adult. At both assessments, he was asked to narrate videoclips that were designed to elicit verbs of motion. Analyses of his narration at 9.5 showed that he was still using a homesign system consistent with what he had used in preschool. As an adult, like other late learners of ASL, his knowledge of ASL grammar was incomplete. This is consistent with research by Newport (1990) who showed that late learners of ASL after 30 years of practice never fully learned ASL grammar, and thus, supports the notion of a critical period in grammatical development. Relevant to the current chapter, though, the accuracy of David's performance depended on the semantic overlap between homesign and ASL. He was able to acquire ASL morphemes whose meanings were the same as his homesign morphemes, but not those that expressed a different meaning. In contrast, the overlap of morpheme forms in homesign and ASL did not affect his performance. Whether the importance of semantic overlap extends to lexical items, as well as morphemes is untested in the literature. It may be that late learners will readily acquire words that are expressed in homesign (e.g., entities and actions) but will have much more difficulty learning words whose referents were not expressed in their homesign system (e.g., abstract concepts).

Research suggests that homesigners replace their homesigns with linguistic signs if they are exposed to sign language prior to adulthood. For instance, Morford (1998) assessed the vocabulary of two adolescent homesigners who were exposed to sign language for the first time at 12 and 13 years of age when they emigrated to the U.S. When asked to label 20 objects and 20 actions, the children used homesigns two months after beginning school, but they used formal signs in this task by the end of two years in school. Emmorey, Grant, and Ewan (1994) documented another homesigner who was first exposed to ASL at 16. She began using signs within 6 weeks of exposure and, after 6 months, over 75% of her lexical items were signs. In addition, adults who learned ASL as a first language in later childhood or adolescence understood signs as shown in research studies on semantic processing (Mayberry & Eichen 1991, described below). Thus, the capacity to acquire the lexicon of a first language extends through adolescence.

For deaf and hard of hearing individuals, this capacity may be limited to acquisition of a sign language. Grimshaw, Adelstein, Bryden and MacKinnon (1998) observed a boy (referred to as E.M.) with a 90db hearing loss who was fitted with hearing aids at 12 years of age that corrected his hearing loss to 35 db. Assessment of his speech as a young adult showed that E.M. still primarily relied on his homesign system and had only acquired a very limited spoken lexicon, leading Grimshaw et al. (1998) to hypothesize that adolescence was past the time for the critical period for acquisition of spoken language. As Grimshaw et al. (1998) and Morford (2003) note, the manual form of homesign may develop the necessary foundations for sign language, but not for spoken language. However, it is impossible to tell if E.M.'s inability to develop a spoken lexicon is due to a critical period for acquisition of the linguistic elements of spoken language or to a critical period, instead, for the ability to process auditory information.

While these case studies show that adolescents learning sign language as their first language can acquire words, consistent with Lenneberg's (1967) original hypotheses, acquisition of a sign lexicon may be much more difficult if exposure occurs after adolescence. In Nicaragua, where sign language use by a Deaf community only began in the late 1970's, many deaf adults were not introduced to sign language until adulthood (referred to as deaf isolates). Kegl, Senghas and Coppola (1999) report that "today, older signers whose repertoire is limited to homesigns are referred to as NO-SABES or 'know nothings,' referring primarily to their inability to acquire Nicaraguan Sign Language" (p. 179). This inability is attributed to the previous linguistic isolation of these adults until past the time of "their critical period for language acquisition" (p. 179). These investigators have documented the inability of these adult learners to acquire the grammar of NSL. Their mastery of a sign lexicon is less well studied. Impressions from communicating with these deaf isolates are that many (but not all) can learn signs. However, the rate of acquisition of words is very slow (Kegl, personal communication, June 13 2004) and it is not clear if these words are learned as linguistic symbols or as unanalyzed wholes (Siple, Caccamise, & Brewer 1982).

This research suggests that late language learners are capable of acquiring a sign lexicon. However, researchers have not examined whether later ages of exposure are related to a reduction in (rather than the absence of) the ability to learn words. Late learners may acquire words at a slower rate. Late learners may need more extensive input or a different type of input (e.g., more explicit instruction) than native or childhood learners to acquire new words. They also may have greater difficulty acquiring words whose referents are not in their homesign system. For instance, after extensive contact with adult Nicaraguan first language learners, Kegl observes that they can acquire signs for things that are concrete and visible but not for more abstract concepts (Kegl, personal communication, June 13 2004).

2.1.2 *Semantic processing*

Mayberry and her colleagues have specifically designed a series of studies to test the critical period hypothesis by examining the effects of age of initial exposure to ASL on adults' ability to process the meaning of sign words (Mayberry 1993; Mayberry & Eichen 1991; Mayberry & Fischer 1989). In these studies, age of exposure was categorized into three levels: infancy (i.e., native signers), childhood (5–8 years old), or adolescence (9–15 years old). Importantly, in all but the initial study (Mayberry & Fischer), the three age-of-exposure groups were matched on length of time they had been using sign language by varying their chronological ages. Thus, practice and age of exposure were not confounded. In addition, the adults had had extensive time to reach linguistic mastery: participants had a minimum of 20 years of sign use, with an average of over 40 years of using ASL as their primary language.

In four different samples of Deaf adults, age of exposure affected the adults' ability to accurately shadow (i.e., verbatim repeating model while viewing) and/or immediately recall (i.e., verbatim signing after model is finished) sign sentences (Mayberry 1993; Mayberry & Eichen 1991; Mayberry & Fischer 1989). Errors, measured by the number of words that were deleted or changed, increased linearly as age of exposure increased, with differences occurring between all four age groups (native, early childhood, elementary school, and adolescents.) In addition, different types of sign substitutions were made by the age of exposure groups. Younger language learners tended to substitute a semantically related sign; that is, their mistakes were clearly related to the meaning of the target signs. For example, some adults produced the word *older* instead of younger for the target sentence *I looked everywhere for my younger brother* (Mayberry 1994:65). In contrast, late language learners were more likely to substitute a phonologically related sign with no semantic or syntactic relationship to the target sign. For example, for the target sentence, *I ate too much turkey and potato at Thanksgiving dinner*, one late learner substituted the sign *sleep* for *and* (Mayberry 1994:67). Although these two signs begin and end with the same handshapes, their place and orientation of articulation differ, resulting in the nonsense sentence *I ate too much turkey sleep potato at Thanksgiving dinner*. These types of errors resulted in different levels of comprehension: Posttest comprehension scores were positively correlated with semantically based errors ($r = +.74$) and negatively correlated with phonologically related errors ($r = -.84$; Mayberry & Fischer 1989). In addition, performance correlated with the adults' self-report of their ability to understand ASL in naturalistic contexts. Semantic processing errors occurred at the lexical level and not merely as a consequence of syntactic deficits. Age of exposure equally affected recall of randomly arranged (ungrammatical) signed sentences, ASL, and Pidgin Sign English sentences. Thus, later acquisition of ASL resulted in difficulties quickly processing the meaning of signs and in understanding sign in everyday conversations due to errors at the lexical level.

Mayberry (1994) concluded that these problems reflected a "phonological bottleneck" in language processing. Because phonological processing is not automatic, later language learners have to engage in effortful processing of the surface, phonological, features of sign words, and therefore have less attention available for accessing the meaning of words. Mayberry pointed out that these late learners had acquired the phonological structure of ASL, since the incorrect signs they produced were close phonologically to the target words. However, she posited that there is a critical period in the development of the ability to use that knowledge when trying to automatically and quickly retrieve word meaning. Even after 40 or 50 years of practice, later learners had not acquired effortless phonological processing. There appears to be a gradual decline in the ability to acquire efficient phonological processing from infancy through adolescence. Other researchers have also found that the age of exposure decreases the speed as well as the accuracy with which signers can access the meaning of familiar signs (Emmorey & Corina 1990; Mayberry & Witcher 2002).

To test the hypothesis that the effects of late learning occurs only for the acquisition of a first language, Mayberry extended her earlier research by comparing semantic processing in adults who became deafened after early childhood and had acquired ASL in adolescence as a second language to three groups of first language learners (Mayberry 1993). All deaf adults had been using ASL as their primary language of communication for an average of 50 years. Performance by these later deafened adults resembled signers who acquired ASL during childhood rather than signers who acquired ASL as a first language during adolescence. In addition, the ability to accurately recall the meaning of sentences was related to age of exposure only for first language learners. Native signers outperformed childhood language learners, who outperformed adolescent first language learners, but adolescent second language learners performed better than childhood first language learners. Thus, learning spoken English early seemed to allow these deaf adults to access the meaning of ASL signs efficiently. In addition, in her earlier study, Mayberry found that the ability of deaf college students who have hearing parents to process ASL signs was related to their receptive spoken (English) vocabulary. These results suggest that what needs to be learned during childhood is not modality specific. Mayberry (1993) suggests that the linguistic skills acquired because of typical early language development would allow these late learners to "bootstrap" or translate the ASL signs to that native language. However, age of exposure effects seem to occur at the very initial stages of processing and thus would not seem to be amenable to conscious bootstrapping. It also might be that the most important effect of early language learning, regardless of mode, is (as Mayberry proposed) the ability to acquire a system of phonology that will, in turn, provide a basis for efficient learning of lexical items. At least some aspects of the formal structural phonological system that are learned in early language acquisition may be amodal. To the degree that basic underlying processes such as phonology are not automatic, the entire process of language learning may be impeded.

Early exposure to a language regardless of modality seems to be necessary to develop the neural bases underlying typical lexical processing. Leybaert and D'Hondt (2003) found that deaf adults who had early exposure to either sign language or cued speech displayed more evidence of left hemisphere specialization when processing single words (signed or cued, depending on native language) than those first exposed to these languages after early childhood. They suggest that the initial bias toward cerebral specialization that exists during infancy requires early linguistic exposure to fully develop, and thus will disappear or be distorted for language-deprived deaf children.

In summary, research provides evidence that access to a first language during early childhood is critical for developing the ability to automatically process the meaning of words. In addition to influencing online comprehension, problems with semantic processing undoubtedly result in difficulty acquiring new words quickly, which will result in slower vocabulary growth. Although research on age of exposure on sign language acquisition has not examined the rate or nature of lexical growth, this issue has been addressed in recent research on the age of exposure by variations in early intervention and cochlear implantation.

2.2 Evidence from timing of intervention during early childhood

Since the 1970s, educational and technological reforms for deaf children who live in industrialized countries have made lack of access to language until after early childhood a rare phenomenon. Therefore, age of exposure is generally earlier than in previous generations of deaf children. This has moved the focus of research relevant to critical periods from the previous focus on a delineation at adolescence to one even earlier – as early as the mid-infancy period (Yoshinaga-Itano, Sedey, Coulter, & Mehl 1998). The trend of earlier identification is accelerating because of current possibilities of identifying hearing loss immediately or soon after birth (Arehart, Yoshinaga-Itano, Thomson, Gabbard, & Stredler-Brown 1998). Because of educational and technological advances, enhanced access to language typically begins soon after the identification of deaf children's hearing loss. Subsequent intervention efforts aim to make language more accessible either by the use of signs and/or by making spoken language perceptible through the use of technologically advanced hearing aids or cochlear implants. The latter has particularly made spoken language dramatically more accessible to deaf children (see Schauwers et al. this volume). Thus, as the age of identification of hearing loss has decreased, so has the age at which most deaf children are provided access to language models. This research suggests that variations of the age of language exposure within the preschool period impact some aspects of semantic development.

2.2.1 *Early identification and intervention*

The hypothesis that the preschool years are a critical period for all types of learning has been advanced since the 1960s, and has served as the impetus for the growth of early intervention for all special needs children (Bailey et al. 2001). For deaf children with hearing parents, identification and intervention is necessary (though not necessarily sufficient) to allow access to auditory and/or sign language input. Research has primarily focused on the effectiveness of early intervention for children's language development (Yoshinaga-Itano et al. 1998). Such effectiveness is assessed by comparing those children who experienced early intervention with those who only received later intervention or by showing that deaf children who received early intervention services were developing language skills approximating or equivalent to those of typically-developing hearing children.

Initial research with deaf children suggested early intervention did not have long-term impact on their language development. For example, in a longitudinal study of all deaf children enrolled in early intervention in Ontario during the mid-1980s, Musselman, Wilson and Lindsay (1988) compared the language and speech skills of children who entered early intervention prior to 24 months with those who entered intervention between 24 and 36 months of age. Earlier intervention resulted in better receptive language but not better expressive language during preschool. However, even this advantage faded by the time the children were in elementary school, with age of intervention not relating to any measure of speech or language skills. At all ages, and for all aspects of language, including vocabulary, these children's language development was severely delayed, suggesting the intervention was not very effective.

More recent research, focusing on earlier ages of identification and intervention, suggests that early intervention can be effective and may need to begin earlier than previously assumed. In ground-breaking work that was the basis for implementing universal newborn screening for hearing loss in the United States and abroad, Yoshinaga-Itano and her colleagues (Mayne, Yoshinaga-Itano, Sedey, & Carey 2000a, 2000b; Yoshinaga-Itano et al. 1998) examined the impact of the timing of early identification and intervention on deaf children's language development for children who were enrolled in an intensive state-wide intervention program (Colorado Home Intervention Program or CHIP). The families of these children used a variety of communication approaches, with some parents choosing to use an oral-only approach, while others using simultaneous communication (sign and spoken English) with their children. In an initial study, general language development was assessed using the parent report instrument Minnesota Communicative Development Inventory when participants were between 13 and 30 months (mean 26 months) of age (Yoshinaga-Itano et al. 1998). Age of identification of hearing loss was divided into four time periods: 0–6; 7–12, 13–18, 19–24, and 25–34 months, with half of the 150 participants being identified before 6 months and from 14 to 25 children identified at each of the other 3 time periods. Median time between identification and intervention was 3 months for these children; thus, enhanced access to language occurred, on average, before 9 months for the early-identified children. Early identification was so effective for facilitating language development that the average performance of these earliest-identified children at preschool age was close to hearing norms. For early-identified children without cognitive delays, language quotients (language age/chronological age) averaged 91, while that for children identified after 6 months averaged 70. The most significant evidence for a critical period for the stimulation of language growth was that language was not affected by differences in age of identification when it occurred after six months; the three groups of later identified children all had equal language quotients. This indicates that time of initial intervention was the critical factor rather than duration of time exposed to intervention. Thus, this study suggests that exposure to language before nine months of age may be a critical period for language development, which at the ages measured here primarily consisted of vocabulary development. This is a much earlier "critical period" than had been proposed in the past.

Subsequent research by the Colorado research team supported the effectiveness of early identification and intervention specifically for vocabulary development with a new sample of children (Mayne et al. 2000a, 2000b). Again the sample included some children whose families were using an oral-only approach and some whose families were using signs. Unlike the earlier study, children were only classified as identified before and after 6 months, with no distinctions within the later identified ages because fewer children were being identified after 6 months due to newborn screening for hearing loss. Mayne et al. (2000a, 2000b) used the MacArthur Communicative Development Inventory (CDI), a parent report instrument, to assess the number of words in children's lexicons when they were between 24 and 37 months old. The researchers found that children who were identified before 6 months had significantly larger lexicons than those identified after 6 months. Only the earlier-identified children, on average, had vocabulary scores that were comparable to their hearing peers, scoring within the 5 to 25 percentile on hearing norms. In addition, normative graphs suggest that early-identified children transitioned from slow to more rapid word learning six months earlier (26 versus 32 months) than later-identified children. In these studies, vocabulary and other aspects of language performance were unrelated to children's degree of hearing loss, mode of communication (sign and spoken English or oral-only), or socio-economic status.

Moeller (2000) also found that an early intervention program based in Omaha, Nebraska, provided effective means of developing age-appropriate vocabulary skills in deaf children with hearing parents. These families were evenly divided between those that used an oral only approach and those that used both spoken and signed English. Both age of intervention and family involvement were predictive of deaf children's vocabulary knowledge at 5 years of age, accounting for 55% of the variance in scores on the Peabody Picture Vocabulary Test. In Moeller's study, age of enrollment in the intervention program ranged from 1–54 months and was divided into four levels for analyses (0–11; 12–23; 24–35; and > 35 months). PPVT scores at age 5 decreased linearly and significantly with increasing age of enrollment. Children whose families were rated as having "ideal" or "good" involvement with their children's education had standard scores comparable to hearing peers. Standard scores averaged from 85 to

100, depending on age of identification. Children whose parents were less involved (average to limited involvement) had smaller lexicons. Standard scores averaged from 60 to 80, depending on age of identification.

These studies provide strong evidence that intensive early intervention prior to 12 months is more effective than similar interventions after the first year in preventing severe language delay for deaf preschoolers, and that close to typical language can occur for early-identified children who do not have cognitive disabilities. Given recent research on the language learning that occurs during the first year of life (e.g., determining word boundaries, learning the phonological categories of language, see Kuhl 2000, for a review), it is not surprising that linguistic input would be required from infancy for age-appropriate language development. However, these studies (Mayne et al. 2000a, 2000b; Moeller 2000) do not show definitively that there is a critical period for vocabulary acquisition. Given the naturalistic approach demanded of such studies, it is not possible to control for all potentially confounding factors. In addition, the designs of both studies confound age of intervention and length of practice. That is, if all children are tested at age 5, those who began intervention services earlier had more intervention time during which to acquire vocabulary. Even if there was not a critical period, language levels should be related to age of intervention, unless later identified children were expected to "catch-up" or experience faster language growth between the time they were identified and the time language was assessed. Only the one result from Yoshinaga-Itano et al. (1998) that found differences between children identified by 6 months and those identified later, and no significant differences among the later age groups is indicative of a critical period. However, research on the development of deaf children using cochlear implants also suggests the possibility of an early critical period.

2.3 Evidence from children with cochlear implants

Since the 1980s many deaf children have had the opportunity to use cochlear implants instead of traditional hearing aids. These implants provide electrical stimulation directly to endings of the auditory nerve, thus bypassing structures in the cochlea (called hair cells) that are frequently damaged in cases of profound hearing loss. The quality of information that is transmitted through use of cochlear implants to neurological centers that process auditory information does not match that received though normal hearing. Input obtained through a cochlear implant has been referred to as "degraded." It is less rich and finely detailed than that received by children without hearing loss (see Schauwers et al. this volume, for a more in-depth description of cochlear implants). Despite this limitation, cochlear implants have given access to sound to many children for whom traditional hearing aids were ineffective. And, because deaf children's access to audition and to spoken language models is usually so deficient before they begin using cochlear implants, their development after obtaining these devices can provide useful information about plasticity – and therefore critical periods – for processing auditory-based language.

It is important to keep in mind before reviewing studies of language development with use of cochlear implants, that research findings are varied, sometimes even contradictory, and any review of existing findings will illuminate difficulties in research design that are typical when outcomes of an essentially clinical program are addressed. One overarching problem is the diversity in pre-language and language experiences of children who are deaf. Some are exposed to sign early in life while others are not. In addition, even profoundly deaf children vary in the degree to which they can detect and discriminate between sounds when using traditional hearing aids. Some can process enough sound so that their auditory pathways are stimulated to some degree before they obtain a cochlear implant, while others are effectively without access to any auditory information. Thus, children would differ on the degree they experience auditory neural growth prior to cochlear implantation. This naturally-occurring complication is exacerbated by differences and even flaws in the research designs that have been employed to track the effects of cochlear implant use. For example, many available studies included such small numbers of participants that any meaningful use of parametric statistical analysis was precluded. In addition, studies frequently lack appropriate comparison groups. Over the past 20-plus years, there have been advances in the technology the cochlear implants employ, thus comparisons across various ages of implant users often include a range of implant effectiveness that is not accounted for in the research design. In addition, the age at which a cochlear implant can be obtained has been changing as both earlier identification of hearing loss and earlier cochlear implantation have appeared to have positive outcomes. Since 2002, the U. S. Food and Drug Administration has approved implantation of profoundly deaf infants at age 12 months and subsequently many children have been implanted between 1 and 2 years of age. There are some exceptions allowing implantation even earlier than 12 months (Geers in press), and a number of infants below 1 year of age have been implanted in the U.S. and other countries. Although this lowering of age at implant has provided opportunities to evaluate age effects, it has complicated interpretation of studies that compare development of children implanted before and after any specific age. For example, if the age break was set at 3 years in older studies, implantation in the younger group probably occurred between 2 and 3 years of age. In more recent studies, the age range in the "below 3" group might well include children implanted as early as 12 months.

A number of reports have indicated advantages for children getting cochlear implants at younger versus older ages on speech perception, general language abilities, and even literacy skills. The age considered "younger" has been variable, however, with some comparing children receiving the implant before and after 5 years, others comparing children receiving implants before and after 3 years, and more recent reports comparing those who received cochlear implants before and after about 2 years of age. It is generally acknowledged, however, that numerous factors, other than age of implantation, affect use of cochlear implants. These factors include but are not limited to nonverbal cognitive skills, history of experience with audition, use of sign or oral-only language, depth of electrode insertion, number of electrodes activated, sophistication of the strategies used by the speech processor component of the cochlear implant device, and family characteristics (Spencer & Marschark 2003). Recent studies have attempted to control for various factors and therefore have begun to provide more specific information about effects of age at implantation.

Connor, Heiber, Arts and Zwolan (2000) conducted a major study of children who received cochlear implants during preschool and elementary school ages. They found that children who received a cochlear implant prior to 5 years of age had higher scores on both receptive and expressive vocabulary measures than those who were not implanted until later, regardless of the language modalities (sign and speech or speech only) they used. Children who received their implants at age 2 showed an average growth rate of .63 years for every year of growth expected for hearing children. The quotient for children receiving their implants at age 6–1/2 was only .45 year of vocabulary growth for every one-year's growth expected from hearing children. These differences appear stable throughout elementary school. Although age of implantation had complex interactions with language mode on some areas of language tested, and effects were also found for technology sophistication, the researchers concluded that earlier implantation had significant effects on vocabulary outcomes.

Connor and Zwolan (in press) further specified effects on vocabulary in a follow-up study focused on reading achievement. In this analysis, both pre-implant vocabulary scores (developed either through sign or oral methods) and age of implantation had effects on post-implant vocabulary. Higher pre-implant vocabulary scores and lower age of implantation both were associated with higher post-implant vocabulary scores. These results point out one of the difficulties with using data on children with cochlear implants to increase understanding regarding a critical period. Although all of the children in this analysis had delayed acquisition of a lexicon, and in most cases the delay would have been quite severe without cochlear implantation, there was some history of development for some of the children. Children who were using signs pre-implant cannot be thought of as having "no" access to language. In fact, Szagun (2001) found that vocabulary scores were related to pre-implant vocabulary knowledge (signed and spoken) but not to age of implantation. In addition, those who had acquired some spoken words probably had some, albeit quite limited, amplified auditory experience pre-implant. Previous auditory experience, whether due to presence of some residual hearing or hearing loss after birth has been found to relate to skills using a cochlear implant (Spencer in press; Szagun 2001).

In order to more clearly use age of cochlear implantation as an indicator of when children gained access to language, Connor and colleagues (Connor, Raudenbush, Zwolan, Heavner, & Craig submitted) conducted a follow-up study examining vocabulary growth rates of children who were in an oral-only environment. Children were divided into three age of implantation groups: 1 to 3.5 years; 3.6 to 7 years; 7.1 to 10 years. Growth curve analysis indicated that children in the first group experienced faster lexical growth than later implanted children for the first two or three years post-implantation. Children who were implanted between 3.6 and 7 years experienced faster growth for one year after implantation compared to children implanted between 7 and 10 years of age. After these initial accelerated learning periods, the trajectory of lexical growth was the same in all three groups, although the higher levels of vocabulary knowledge due to the earlier "bursts" were maintained. In other words, although the initial advantage of having an earlier implantation does not result in faster lexical growth throughout childhood, there is a permanent effect on the level of vocabulary knowledge at least through elementary school. In fact, the rate of growth for the earlier implanted oral children approximated that expected for hearing children. These results suggest a heightened sensitivity to spoken language input prior to age 3.5, with a gradual (though not absent) decline in sensitivity from 3.5 to 7 years.

Recent reports have suggested even earlier critical periods or "break points" for initial access to auditory-based language through use of cochlear implants. Based on the MacArthur Communicative Development Inventory (CDI), Svirsky, Teoh and Neuberger (in press) found accelerated acquisition of vocabulary for children implanted between 12 and 24 months compared with those implanted at or after 25 months. Similarly Kirk, Miyamoto, Lento, Ying, O'Neill and Fears (2002) reported faster rates of acquisition for children less than two years old at time of implant compared to those implanted between two and three years.

Using the PPVT-III to test receptive vocabulary plus analysis of a spontaneous language sample, Nicholas and Geers (2003, in press) found evidence of age effects even below 2 years of age. They found that children implanted before 19 months of age acquired lexical items at a rate near that expected for hearing children. Children receiving implants between 19 and 24 months showed somewhat slower vocabulary acquisition. Those receiving implants after 24 months of age were even more delayed. In this study, all children were assessed at the age of 3.5 years, so duration of cochlear implant use differed. Nicholas and Geers (in press) in a review of existing literature on the outcomes of early cochlear implantation, proposed that the age of two years might mark the end of a critical period for support of "normal" rates of language (and vocabulary) learning.

Support for a critical period for lexical development is not unequivocal. Although age of acquisition has consistently affected syntactic growth, several studies have not found a relationship between age of implantation and vocabulary measures (Dawson, Blamey, Dettman, Barker, & Clark 1995b; Spencer in press; Szagun 2001). Despite these few contradictory findings, the more recent studies indicate early implantation results in better vocabulary development across some age levels. However, other factors (e.g., pre-implant vocabulary, pre-implant auditory experience) also have significant effects. Because so many varied age "breaks" have been suggested, and because those currently being indicated fall within ages posited to encompass a critical period for auditory processing itself, it is difficult to attribute direct effects of age of language exposure on vocabulary. Such apparent effects may be due to the impact of early exposure to sound on auditory processing which leads to efficient phonological processing and indirectly results in advantaged patterns of lexical acquisition (Connor et al. submitted).

3. Critical periods and word learning processes

The influence of age of exposure on lexical growth rate may be due to differences in children's word learning processes. One of the most amazing feats of typical lexical development is the ability of hearing children to acquire as many as eight new words a day (Golinkoff, Hirsh-Pasek, Bloom, Smith, Woodward,

Akhtar, Tomasello, & Hollich 2000). This ability depends on hearing children's ability to fast map, or store an initial meaning of a new word after only a few exposures. Rather than needing explicit instruction, children can fast map new words incidentally by using contextual cues to derive meaning. By varying the context that novel (usually nonsense or nonce) words are used, researchers have established that hearing two- and three-year-olds can use a variety of social, cognitive, and linguistic cues to fast map the meaning of new words (Golinkoff et al. 2002).

Do deaf children also develop these skills and does their development show critical period effects? Lederberg and Spencer examined fast mapping in deaf preschoolers by assessing their ability to quickly learn an initial meaning of nonce words presented to them in two different contexts (Lederberg, Prezbindowski, & Spencer 2000; Lederberg & Spencer 2001). The tasks were designed to isolate the cognitive aspects of fast mapping as much as possible. Word learning was assessed by testing the children's comprehension of the meaning of the new words, rather than production. The nonce words were phonologically simple and easily distinguishable from words that were likely to be part of the children's lexicon; spoken nonce words consisted of either one or two syllables (e.g., *dax*, *nupa*); sign words were structurally simple and used handshapes, location and direction/orientation of movement that are consistent with citation signs in both ASL and English signing systems. Depending on individual children's language learning environments, the tasks were either conducted in simultaneous (sign and spoken) communication or speech alone. The tasks also used a "naming game" structure that minimized the attentional demands for the children and made clear the task was to learn new words. Two levels of fast mapping abilities were assessed. In one, the meanings of nonce words were made clear by the researcher through explicit social and pragmatic clues (i.e., pointing and/or holding a novel object while saying/signing *nupa*). In the second, implicit, context, children had to infer that the nonce words referred to novel objects in the absence of social/pragmatic cues; that is decide that dax referred to a novel object such as a garlic press rather than to shoe, dog, or chair. The 100 deaf and hard of hearing preschoolers tested had gained access to linguistic input from birth through four years of age and included children in both oral and simultaneous communication environments. The development of these word learning abilities was primarily associated with the size of the children's lexicon, rather than their chronological age. Children who were in the initial stages of vocabulary development (as measured by the number of words they produced) did not learn words in either context. Thus, these children did not fastmap words. Children with moderately-sized lexicons learned nonce words but only when the meaning of a word was made explicit by social and pragmatic cues. Finally, those children with larger lexicons were also able to infer the meaning of words by the context.

Longitudinal research showed that acquisition of these word learning processes was linked to the growth of a larger lexicon (Lederberg et al. 2000; Lederberg, Spencer, & Huston 2003). In other words, as children acquired more words, they also acquired these word learning processes. Relations between lexicon size and the word learning processes were the same for children acquiring spoken or sign language, those with a cochlear implant and those without, and for children who ranged in age of exposure to accessible input from birth to 4 years of age. Acquisition of the processes ranged from two to 6 years of age. Thus, there does not appear to be a critical period for the acquisition of fastmapping, at least if age of exposure occurs during the preschool years. However, because of the link between fastmapping and lexicon size, factors that affect vocabulary growth will also affect how quickly the processes are acquired.

Although young children learn words from conversational context, for older children learning of new words frequently occurs in the reading context. De Villiers and Pomerantz (1992) examined the ability of middle and high school deaf and hard of hearing students to infer the meaning of new words from reading them in a short narrative passage that contained cues to the words' meanings. Children from both oral and simultaneous communications language environments were included in the study. Students at both ages and language environments were able to learn an initial meaning for some of the words from reading the passage once, although better readers were able to fast map more words than poorer readers. This suggests that if children were able to understand the semantic, contextual cues given in these passages, they were able to infer the meaning of the words. Although the researchers did not report the age these children gained access to language, given that the cohort of children were born during the 1970s, it is likely most of them gained access to language ranging in age between 2 and 6 years old. Thus, again, there did not appear to be a critical period for the acquisition of cognitively based word learning processes (the ability to learn the meaning of new words from context). On the other hand, acquisition of the grammatical nature of the new words did not occur during the fast mapping process. Even though the children could assign meaning to words, they could not infer their form class from the reading context. Specifically, they could not categorize the words as nouns, verbs, or adjectives nor could they make judgments about the words' correct syntactic usages.

Establishing the meaning and grammatical information of new words from contextual cues is not the only process involved in learning new words. Learning new words also depends on children's ability to represent or encode the phonological structure of words, and the latter may be a source of slower lexical growth. Gilbertson and Kamhi (1995) studied elementary school children's word learning processes by assessing the ability to both comprehend the meaning of nonce words and to accurately produce the words after only a few exposures. To examine the effect of the phonological structure on learning, the nonce words varied in complexity (specifically *tam*, *jaften*, *shabaffidy*, *gadakik*). Participants were hearing children and hard of hearing (rather than deaf) children who were mainstreamed in school. Consistent with past research, hard of hearing children had no problems fast mapping the meaning of the nonce words, with no effect of phonological structure on comprehension. The hearing children and half of the hard of hearing children were also able to accurately produce the words after only four exposures. These hard of hearing children also performed within typical age limits on standardized tests of receptive and expressive vocabulary. In contrast, half of the hard of hearing children had much more difficulty learning to produce the two complex words, sometimes not producing them correctly even after 10 exposures. These latter children performed well below age norms on standardized tests of both receptive and expressive vocabulary. In other words, the children who had difficulty producing the new words had much smaller vocabularies. Thus, this research suggests slower lexical growth may be caused by the speed children can represent and produce the correct phonological structure, rather than the meaning, of new words. Although this study did not examine the effect of age of exposure on word learning processes, it points to a mechanism in which age of acquisition effects on phonological processing could result in slower lexical acquisition.

4. Conclusions

Research with deaf individuals supports the conclusion that there is no critical period for acquisition for some aspects of lexical development, at least if that exposure occurs before adulthood, and if that language is visual. Late learners of sign language are able to acquire a sign lexicon (Mayberry 1994). This may be due, in part, to the fact that children acquire some foundational skills through the development of nonlinguistic homesign communication systems (Goldin-Meadow 2003). Even without access to language, children develop the ability to use nonlinguistic gestural symbols to refer to the aspects of their environment usually labeled by nouns, verbs, and adjectives. Homesigns refer to categories of referents and can have multiple meanings. Finally, children acquire both conventional gestures that have a stable form and meaning, and gestures that have a simple sublexical morphological-like (but probably not phonological) structure. At least through adolescence (and maybe longer), homesigners seem to be able to transfer these skills to the acquisition of a linguistic, sign, lexicon.

Acquisition of some word learning processes that establish meaning or reference for words also seem to be robust to differences in age of exposure, although this research has only explored variations from birth through five years of age (de Villiers & Pomerantz 1992; Lederberg et al. 2000). Once children have acquired a lexicon of sufficient size, they develop word learning processes that allow them to fast map an initial meaning of new words using contextual cues. These abilities depend on level of vocabulary development rather than the age that vocabulary development began.

On the other hand, age of exposure seems to affect lexical growth rate. Although more research is needed, research on the effects of early intervention and on effects of cochlear implantation suggest that lexical growth is faster for children exposed to language by one or two years of age than for those with later language exposures (Connor et al. submitted; Kirk et al. 2002; Mayne et al. 2000a; Nicholas & Geers in press; Svirsky et al. in press). Current findings are clearly insufficient to determine the exact timing and shape of this critical period. While some findings suggest growth rate declines rapidly after these ages, other research shows a more gradual, continuous, decline throughout childhood (Connor et al. 2000; Connor et al. submitted).

There also seems to be a critical period for ultimate attainment of efficient and automatic semantic processing. Later language exposure results in difficulty quickly and accurately understanding the meaning of familiar words, even after 40 years of language use (Emmorey & Corina 1990; Mayberry 1994). Comprehension abilities appear to be related to age of exposure, with understanding declining as age of exposure increased from birth to childhood to adolescence.

What underlies these critical period effects? Some researchers suggest the critical period effects are caused by the permanent deleterious effects of auditory deprivation on auditory processing (Connor et al. submitted). Indeed, Sharma, Dorman and Spohr (2002a, 2002b) found age of cochlear implantation effects on cortical auditory-evoked response waveform, with implantation by 3.5 years of age necessary for the development of typical cortical level auditory processing mechanisms. Children implanted after 3.5 were much less likely to show normalized PI latencies. Earlier access to sound through cochlear implantation, hearing aids, and auditory-based interventions seems to result in better development of the auditory neural pathways. Better auditory processing facilitates quick and efficient encoding of phonemes of spoken words and thus quicker lexical growth.

Although undoubtedly true, critical period effects are not exclusively accountable by auditory development, since evidence for critical period effects on lexical growth, semantic processing, and cerebral laterialization for language processing have been found for deaf individuals using sign language or cued speech (Leybaert & D'Hondt 2003; Mayberry 1994; Mayne et al. 2000a). Given that homesigners develop a visual representational system, the problem is not one of sensory deprivation or delayed representational skills. In addition, since this effect is evident for children acquiring speech, sign, and cued speech, it is not specific to a certain type of linguistic representation. Mayberry argues lexical skills depend on the efficiency of the phonological system. Timing of language exposure may have permanent effects on the degree to which the processing and encoding of the phonological structure of words is efficient and automatic (Ruben 1997), which in turn, affects lexical growth and semantic processing. Mayberry's research on second language learning raises the intriguing possibility that such effects are amodal (Mayberry 1993). In other words, the critical period may be for exposure and learning a phonological system from early exposure to either sign or spoken words, and such learning would allow the later acquisition of a sign or spoken language (provided there are no auditory deprivation effects). Connor and Zwolan's (in press) finding that preimplant (sign) vocabulary is related to postimplant lexical knowledge is also consistent with the hypothesis that very early exposure and knowledge of a phonological system has long-lasting effects on lexical development, regardless of modality.

Finally, although the process of inferring meaning from context for new words may be robust; it relies on the ability to understand the contextual cues to that meaning. Clearly, if later exposure to language results in poorer semantic processing or reading abilities, lexical growth may be slower as a consequence of later learners' lack of understanding of the context of new words (de Villiers & Pomerantz 1992). In addition, poorer syntactic skills resulting from later exposure to language would interfere with word learning based on the syntactic form of new words, something that hearing children use from a very young age. For example, hearing toddlers use the following syntactic frames to differentiate possible meanings of a novel word: "Here is a bipi." "Here is bipi." "Here is some bipi." (Golinkoff et al. 2000). Thus, if critical period results in poorer syntactic processing, it will also result in slower lexical growth.

In summary, this research review suggests that there is a critical period for some aspects of semantic development. Current trends toward earlier identification of hearing loss with the result of earlier provision of accessible language models to deaf children, through signing and/or amplification or cochlear implants, will undoubtedly provide additional information relevant to this issue. We believe that investigations of the nature and rate of lexical development and of word learning processes may shed further light on the issue of a critical period for the ease with which vocabulary is acquired over the life span.

Developmental theory and language disorders

A thematic summary

Michael Garman, Deborah James and Vesna Stojanovik

1. Introduction

We have in this collection a wide range of state-of-the-art reviews of language disorders that are informed by developmental theory, and brought together conveniently in a single volume. They allow us the opportunity to draw things together, identify where productive links are possible, where gaps need filling, and keep taking us back to the fundamental nature of language disorders and of the language development process itself. Miller (1983) referred to the distinction between (1) the traditional aetiological approach, in terms of which "children are first sorted out according to the condition thought to be the *cause* of the language disorder" and (2) the newer approach by which "children are first sorted out by the *consequences*, or the presenting symptoms, of the language disorder". Leonard (1983) expanded this to include (3) "the intervention-linked model" by which "children are sorted according to characteristics that have a bearing on the choice of language intervention procedures to use with a child."

Within this framework, twenty years of research have addressed the fuller development of each approach, and the current volume provides a status report on this large enterprise. It is clear that important advances have been made: in their introduction, Miller and Fletcher note that the behavioral classification of mental retardation in the 1980s reflected the fact that 30% of children had an identified aetiology, whereas now the figure is more like 80%. At the same time, considerable advances have been made in improving the quality of the behavioral evidence over the range of disorders, although more still needs to be done in this regard, e.g. in improving our knowledge of what sort of language abilities are to be expected for a given type or level of mental retardation. A number of contributors also address the clinical or intervention implications of current research. In this area, the sense of optimism that is rightly generated by particular insights is tempered by blunt questions such as (Miller & Fletcher) "Why do SLI children fail to grow out of their problems?". Similarly, Thomas asks, if there is compensation among the interacting levels in the language processing system, why is there no recovery of genetic developmental language disorders as there is of disorders associated with early focal lesions? And there is evidence that, as some children with specific language impairment grow up, they show increasingly autistic-type behavior (Gernsbacher, Geye, & Weismer). The two sides of the issue are captured in the observation that with a cochlear implant (CI), deaf children may show a normal rate of subsequent language development, but, depending on the age of CI, this is from a lower base, and any language delay may not be eradicated (Schauwers, Gillis, & Govaerts; Lederberg & Spencer).

It is striking how the research reported in this volume seeks to keep the first two approaches in balance: where there is better description, let there be also greater causal understanding; where there is greater certainty about identified cause, let us know still more about how it can be manifested. There is, then, no sense of a reductionist stance in the relation between these approaches. However, it would not be too distorting to see the development of the third approach as the ultimate rationale for this research field – the prospect of effective intervention not only improves quality of life for the individuals concerned but also constitutes our best guarantee of our understanding of how language fits with our other cognitive abilities, in development and beyond.

Most of the language disorders addressed in this volume may be characterized very generally as developmental, although there are great differences between them. There are those that have a genetic basis for mental retardation (MR), within which aspects of language development are impacted:

Down Syndrome (DS): Abbeduto and Chapman; Gernsbacher et al.

Fragile X Syndrome (FraXS): Abbeduto and Chapman

Williams Syndrome (WS): Thomas; Gernsbacher et al.

There are those that have been variously thought to have a basis in social/emotional impairment, psycholinguistic processing, pragmatics or social cognition:

Autism: Gernsbacher et al.
Asperger's Disorder: Gernsbacher et al.

There is the situation where an otherwise functional language and cognitive ability develops without typical exposure to language:

Hearing Impairment (HI): Schauwers et al.; Lederberg and Spencer

And there are those types of language disorder which have been identified principally on behavioral evidence, and whose causal origins are currently obscure (probably lying within, or very closely associated to, mechanisms or processes that are specific to, or crucially involved in, language):

Specific Language Impairment (SLI): Thomas; Fletcher, Stokes and Wong; Gernsbacher et al.

Pragmatic Language Impairment: Gernsbacher et al.

Specific Language Delay: Gernsbacher et al.

And finally we have the case where typical childhood milestones are interrupted and regressed by epileptiform EEG abnormalities:

Landau-Kleffner Syndrome (LKS): Gernsbacher et al.

The last mentioned case brings us to the consideration of the distinction between developmental and acquired disorders. It may be sharply drawn in terms of aetiology, e.g., in cases where focal brain injury is a clear cause of language disorder in an otherwise typical course of childhood development; but even in these cases, establishing the behavioral profile and the approach to intervention will be informed by developmental considerations. In other cases, the sudden emergence of a language-disordering factor may raise the issue of how far the developmental trajectory has really been typical up to that point. Nevertheless, it seems useful to us to draw a distinction between the concept of developmental and acquired language disorders in childhood, and to restrict the term *childhood aphasia* to the non-developmental types.

We may note here that the study of aphasia in adults has seemingly had the benefit of an impressive taxonomy of syndromes and their interrelationships over decades of work; and by comparison, research on child language disorders has seemed to struggle with anything much more sophisticated than the distinction between those children that are impaired in both expressive and receptive language vs. those that are impaired in receptive language only. Rapin and Wilson (1978) noted that "the child neurologist who studies developmental language disability will not encounter the relatively clear syndromes seen in adult aphasics" (p. 24). However, given the qualms that have been expressed over the last few decades re the distorting tendency of aphasic syndromes (Caplan 1987), in the face of considerable individual variation, we might wonder whether child language impairment researchers have not had the better of it, after all. Much constructive groundwork towards an adequate understanding of language impairment is documented in this volume and, while it is clear that much work has still to be done, arguably it is an advantage not to have to engage in too much demolition of unwanted conceptual frameworks beforehand.

Nevertheless, syndromes in childhood language impairment have been recognized, and show their expected attendant issues of interpretation. We find a direct reflection of a principal concern with aphasia syndromes in the observation (Miller & Fletcher) of how difficult it is to find SLI children that fit the accepted definition of the disorder. Gernsbacher et al. note the distinction between the *distinct category* vs. the *dimensional account* and issues arising: How far may individuals be reclassified from one diagnosis to another? How far do syndromes overlap? How far might clients exhibit co-morbidity? How far might syndrome shifts reflect developmental logic?

In this review, our comments are not organized chapter by chapter, but will focus instead on issues that arise across the individual contributions. We shall be selective, and try to address those issues that are, on this evidence, of most general application. First, we have some remarks on the setting for research on language disorders and language development.

2. A framework for language disorders and developmental theory

A convenient framework may be sketched as having three reference points/areas of knowledge, in mutual relationship with each other, as follows:

1. Normal child language development – addressing issues such as,

   stages of language development;
   the contribution of internal and external variables;
   the differential contribution of linguistic vs. cognitive domains;

2. Language disorders – everything in (1) plus the approaches mentioned earlier, namely,

   identifying aetiology;
   documenting behavioral patterns of strength/weakness over time;
   establishing effective intervention;

3. Let us call this reference point something like *mode* (of language performance) – having to do with the scale, extent or nature of the evidence base – ranging over at least the following,

   mono-lingual to cross-linguistic development;
   spoken vs. written media, and sign vs. oral;
   language development vs. mature language use;
   language processes vs. linguistic structures;
   comprehension vs. production;
   variation: this refers to not just individual differences, but also finer within-individual differences over development, as well as more general variation between *styles* of language development. One of the valuable functions of a volume such as the present one is to address the variation within and between different patterns of language disorder.

Between (1) and (2), there has been a long and honorable association, at least since the shift to language (MLU)-based comparisons (Miller & Fletcher; Fletcher et al.). It was a real advance when language delay was established as overwhelmingly more important than language *deviance*, in understanding language disorders, and the benefits have flowed to both fields. However, the distinction is important enough to be continuously tested, and this in turn tests our understanding of the limits of normal variation.

As for (1) and (3), there has been the long-acknowledged need for broadening the evidence base away from monolingual and Anglo-centric studies. Cross-linguistic research is fertile ground for study of normal CLD, particularly in the case of bilingual children. Study of these individuals allows the investigation of cross-linguistic factors under the simultaneous control of cognitive stage of development and of the socioeconomic and family factors that Miller and Fletcher refer to in their introductory chapter. Two earlier TiLAR volumes have concentrated on bilingualism and sign language, and it is appropriate that these areas are not to the fore in the present volume: but it is significant that Lederberg and Spencer provide a careful treatment of sign development, both untutored *homesign* as well as conventional sign language, in pursuit of evidence for critical periods of exposure to language in hearing-impaired children possessing functional language and cognitive ability.

Of the relation between (2) and (3) we can say there is an acknowledged need, and some particular success, but generally much less has been achieved. There is considerable potential for cross-linguistic studies of language disorder, and we may see two types of evidence arising: one from languages that are related in such a way that one can act as a control for some specific factor, e.g. in morphological richness (Leonard 1992); and another, exemplified in Fletcher et al., in which we get a glimpse of what some broad category such as SLI might look like in the very different circumstances of a language such as Cantonese.

There is also the possibility of modality-specific disorder (e.g. Nespoulous 1999), in which might be found an analogy to the use of bilingual children in the crosslinguistic study of language development, thus allowing for control of other factors. This in turn touches on the relation between spoken and written language: how do children with spoken language disorder cope with literacy when they go to school? Gernsbacher et al. refer to the possibility of a "natural category" for dyslexia in school-age children, vs. the lack of such for SLI. Experience over the past 30 years in the Linguistic Assessment Clinic at Reading suggests a fundamental distinction among children who have worked through preschool language impairment, between those for whom the encounter with the written form of English at school represents a further hurdle, and those for whom written English seems to represent a utilizable alternative source of input which can be used to scaffold further language development.

3. Issues

3.1 Similarities and differences, in normal and atypical language development

It is striking that a number of contributors to this volume note commonalities between particular patterns of impaired and normal language development (Thomas; Fletcher et al.; Gernsbacher et al.). This immediately raises the question as to how much we know of normal child language, and as Fletcher et al. point out, this is partly a matter of knowing how to set the level of representation, for a given stage of development. We also have acknowledgement that some disorder patterns such as FraX are not sufficiently well described yet in terms of their general development and language characteristics for the issue of commonality to be determined (Abbeduto & Chapman); or that particular aspects need further investigation, such as fast-mapping abilities in Autism (Gernsbacher et al.).

For the rest of the picture, three main patterns emerge: (a) the presence of uneven profiles within disorders across components of language, and as between language and mental age (MA) (Thomas), which challenge our understanding of the limits of such variation in apparently normal language development; (b) wide variation between individuals within patterns of disorder such as DS, Autism (Abbeduto & Chapman; Gernsbacher et al.), and deaf children who receive cochlear implants (CI), in terms of age, audiological status and exposure to language, reflecting the native language of the parents (i.e., sign or spoken) (Schauwers et al.; Lederberg & Spencer); and (c) overlaps in individuals as between one disorder and another, e.g. Autism/SLI, both in terms of familial as well as behavioral measures (Gernsbacher et al.).

3.2 Partitions and relations in the language system: Lexicon vs. syntax

3.2.1 *The boundary between lexicon and syntax*

For much of the recent period of research in child language, the goal of acquisition has been cast in terms of a sound (or sign)-to-meaning mapping set out in terms of phonetics-phonology, vocabulary, syntax and semantics-pragmatics. This sequence of modules is reflected in terms of standard assessment procedures, in which morpho-syntax abilities are rather distinctly handled in e.g. the TROG (Bishop 1989) from lexical-semantic abilities in the BPVS (Dunn, Dunn, Whetton, & Burley 1997). However, there is a problem in fitting *vocabulary* in this sequence, since it parallels syntax in mediating its own links between sound and meaning. This underlines a fundamental parallelism of two distinct routes mediating sound and meaning – the one via the lexicon, consisting of stored forms that can be retrieved from long term memory, and the other via a computational system of rules that can be implemented on previously unencountered forms of language. In these terms, a child *has language* as soon as he or she meets the conditions of true symbolic function, at the one-word stage (a traditional view) and what subsequently develops is the working out of the implications, for the sound system, for syntax and for semantics. For the sound system, the prelexical period of development which sees the acquisition of sounds as such, is seen as distinct from the postlexical, and the latter is characterized rather as the fast-mapping of word-sized novel and complex sound shapes and the successive analysis of them in terms of recurring contrastive syllable and sub-syllable units. Sounds emerge from words. For adults, too, the serial account of signal processing in terms of a prelexical phonemic code (sounds are perceived as a way to identifying words) has been complemented by one that is essentially word-oriented (words are accessed, and their sound structure becomes available).

For syntax, Fletcher et al. note the grammar-centered approaches to language structure, language development and language assessment and the changing conception of the lexicon vs. syntax up to the development of construction theory, in which there is a continuum between the two, and thus an alternative interpretation of the relation between lexical and syntactic aspects of behavior. Lexical learning carries constructional implications (words, by virtue of their meaning, may take certain arguments), and the acquisition of certain structures may be limited early on to certain words only. What is observed in early child expressive speech or understanding may be simultaneously structure-rich (in the traditional view of holophrases like *up!* carrying whole sentence meaning) and word-limited (in the sense of two-word utterances literally being Word 1 + Word 2, rather than Subject + Verb). Under this outer behavioral level, ongoing word acquisition, and the generalizations thus enabled, support increasingly abstract internal representations of syntax.

3.2.2 *Vocabulary in language disorders*

However, in the main the traditional perspective on the syntax/lexicon boundary remains strong in the study of both typical and atypical language development. For an insight into the central position of vocabulary development with respect to issues in child language, it is instructive to consider the scope of Bloom's (2000) treatment of word learning, as involving "cognitive capacities of considerable richness ... [which] include the ability to learn and store arbitrary mappings..., theory of mind ..., an understanding of concepts corresponding to kinds and individuals ..., and, at least for some words, an appreciation of syntactic cues to meaning" (p. 259).

As vocabulary is the earliest system of signal-to-meaning relations to develop, it is of particular importance to the identification and interpretation of developmental disorders. Its significance is further increased because a lexicon is a system in which "information ... can be accessed efficiently in a number of different ways" (Forster 1976). Further, its own developmental dynamics are compelling: a number of the contributors to this volume note the astonishing rapidity of normal word acquisition, which must be conservatively set at around 8–10 words per day on average, from age 1 to 20 years in the life of the individual. The immediate qualification, that we are surely not dealing here with a constant rate of development, only deepens our interest, as we consider instead a curve that varies from the remarkable to the truly spectacular. The little we directly know of the quantitative dynamics of children's linguistic output, e.g. Wagner's (1985) figures on how much children say in a day, is suggestive of where the upper bounds of lexical performance may lie. Greater knowledge is centered around concepts such as the *vocabulary spurt*, which lies just after the relatively gentle slope of initial vocabulary development (a few words per week), and is associated with the transition between the single-word stage and the onset of multiword utterances, typically around the middle of the second year. Yet even here, the rates reported for the spurt are well below those for vocabulary development as a whole. Also, while the spurt has been a well-attested phenomenon in the literature, Clark (2002) discusses the variation that has been noted regarding its timing and definition, and its absence in some children; and Bloom (2000) is frankly skeptical.

Since Carey and Bartlett's (1978) study, fast mapping of novel words has been recognized as another ability linked to rapid word acquisition in the normal child, and it too is mentioned by a number of contributors. Clearly, the process is itself in need of explanation, since it involves the child's ability to make inferences about possible meanings intended by the other speaker, down to first-pass storage of phonological word shapes. Studies of such abilities reveal, as in many other aspects of vocabulary development, clear asymmetries in which word production lags well behind the development of word comprehension, an area which is still much less well understood.

What is clear, concerning the rate of vocabulary development generally, is that it is not best understood in terms of the accumulation of individual word-units: increasing numbers of words are the end result but they grow as a result of processes that act across the board, providing better lexical representations, in terms of phonology, grammatical deployment, and semantics and conceptual development, for whole areas of vocabulary. What this means is that vocabulary is a multi-faceted construct (Lederberg & Spencer), and while it may be numerically either restricted (as Abbeduto & Chapman report for DS pre-school and childhood periods) or large (as Thomas reports for a number of WS children), it may be underspecified in certain domains. Thus Thomas suggests that vocabulary development in Autism might be affected by interactive links from pragmatic impairment; and Gernsbacher et al. recommend investigation of fast mapping (FM) in Autism, as has been done for normal, DS, WS and SLI populations, and specifically point to the link between lexical and grammatical abilities as an area that needs further investigation in Autism. Thomas also notes that, while WS vocabulary is often relatively strong in lexical semantics, it exhibits weakness in spatio-temporal terms, and in ways that affect morphological marking of specific semantic functions, and is an area of specific anomalies, characterized by imprecise knowledge of concepts and atypical vocabulary usage. He also notes an imbalance between a larger than normal productive vocabulary in relation to comprehension.

3.3 Partitions and relations in the language system: Phonology vs. lexicon and syntax

As well as being assessed in their own terms, deficits in the sound system have long been seen (Tallal & Piercy 1978) as potentially damaging to the development of the larger linguistic system. Thomas notes that phonological impairment itself may originate in low-level auditory processing problems, and that the pathway from phonology to syntax is obscure. He refers to Chiat's (2001) interpretation of SLI arising from impaired phonological processing and consequent impaired mapping between sound and meaning, and asks whether, since phonological problems are not reported for SLI in adulthood, an early stage might have gone unreported? For WS, he notes that phonology shows an initial delay, then develops into the normal range. His modeling analysis shows that manipulations to phonology alone, or to the integration of phonology and semantics, simulated the pattern of WS past tense data.

Abbeduto and Chapman report DS phonological problems as evolving over the lifespan, with infants showing slow transition from babbling to speech and poor intelligibility; childhood characterized by a longer than normal period of phonological errors and greater variability, with intelligibility problems; adolescence still with concerns about intelligibility, and with variable F0, rate, stress; and adulthood with hypernasality, stuttering, and improved intelligibility. Do these problems amount to what Tallal and Piercy (1978) called "a concomitant of the linguistic defect but not causally related to it"?

Schauwers et al. summarize the findings on what is typical of deaf speech: initially, late onset, and delayed development by up to 15–18m, with a low ratio of babbling; a restricted inventory, with a preference for (visible) labials over other places, and for (resonant) nasals over other manners and heavy neutralization of vowels. Later phonological development is characterized by a reduced inventory, with consonant errors: omissions especially in word-final position, place of articulation errors, nasal substitution, vowel errors, especially with high tongue positions; phonological processes include omissions, tense-lax substitutions, vowel monophthongs for diphthongs, and vowel neutralization. Intelligibility shows great variation, linked to the degree of HI – average is 20% of normal, with a range of 0–80%

A question in all this is what effect if any, such documented persistent phonological difficulties have on the emergence of the language system? Thomas notes that children with mild HI exhibit phonological problems without the inflectional morphology problems that are observed in SLI. The picture regarding phonological development in autism is especially intriguing.

Gernsbacher et al.'s review of Kanner's original children is suggestive of subgroups with or without difficulty with early vocabulary. This raises the question what the early phonological development in each of these groups might have been like. Wolk and colleagues (Wolk & Edwards 1993; Wolk & Giesen 2000) have carried out detailed investigations of children with autism and found evidence of delayed phonology, with some atypical patterns. The features they report include restricted use of contrasts, absence of certain sounds (fricatives, affricates and /r/), persistence of labialization, cluster reduction, final consonant deletion, unusual sound changes e.g. glottal replacement and extensive segment coalescence, frication of liquids, velorization, and chronological imbalance of age-appropriate with immature elements. They note a contrast with previous research suggesting delayed rather than unusual phonological development. Tjus, Heimann and Nelson (1998) reported measures of phonological awareness and reading in a treatment study of 13 autistic children that observed gains in reading, phonology and language development. A phonological reflection of social influences is reported in Baron-Cohen and Staunton's (1994) finding that English autistic children of non-English mothers tended, unlike normal controls, to acquire their mother's non-English accent. Finally, McCann and Peppé (2003) provide a literature review of the under-researched area of prosody in autism, reporting conflicting methodologies and findings, and make recommendations for future research.

3.4 Modular vs. interactive accounts

Since Fodor's (1983) landmark study of modularity in language vehement debates in language acquisition research have thrived. While the details of Fodor's proposal have frequently been challenged, e.g. the impenetrability of the internal processing of modules (Marshall 1984), and the encapsulation of modules and the nature of their shallow output (Jackendoff 2000), there seems to be little doubt that the adult brain presents with a modular architecture. As a result, the topic of modularity is unavoidable at any language acquisition forum and the profiles of atypical populations, such as Williams Syndrome, Down Syndrome and Fragile-X Syndrome and Autism, are very much in the spotlight of the debate. What can such profiles tell us about the role of modularity in the development of the language system? The two papers in this volume that consider this issue conclude, on different grounds, that modularity does not provide an adequate explanatory framework to accommodate the commonalities and dissociations observed in atypical language development.

Thomas outlines what is often referred to as *innate modularity*, as represented by those who claim that that modular system observed in the adult is also present in the infant brain so that language development proceeds although one or more components of this system may be anomalous. An alternative framework, referred to as *neuroconstructivism* is based on the premise that the modular structure observed in the adult state is not present in the infant and that modular structure emerges through development. In each case there is a problem in identifying the precise nature of the early system. Thomas takes Williams Syndrome as an example: although research on WS has moved substantially from the initial claims that these children have intact language abilities despite severe cognitive deficits, the emerging picture is much less clear and the question of what WS can tell us about the constraints guiding typical language acquisition is more open than ever before. What seemed initially (when research on WS began in the 1980s) to be the answer to the question of what the underlying mechanisms of language acquisition are has turned into a minefield of highly problematic issues. For the modular account, it is problematic that there is fractionation within modules such as syntax, lexicon and pragmatics, as well as unevenness between them.

Despite the fact that a number of hypotheses have been put forward to explain the uneven language profile observed in WS, it is still very much an open question as to what this population tells us about the constraints guiding typical language acquisition. Computational modeling has been proposed as a more precise way of exploring how sources of information interact in the acquisition of a particular language domain. And although it is powerful enough to challenge the views which postulate domain-specific fractionation (for example, the connectionist past tense model is able to simulate the same behavioral data as found in children with SLI – van der Lely & Ullman 1996) it has a number of limitations: modeling simplifies to a great degree the processes involved in child language acquisition, and so far, it has focused on individual domains only (lexical segmentation, vocabulary acquisition, inflectional morphology, syntax processing rather than the operation of multi-component systems).

Abbeduto and Chapman contrast the modularity account with the social-interactionist view, on two main aspects: strong innate constraints on, and autonomy of, language development vs. intimate bidirectional influences between language and other domains; and a restricted vs. a critical role for experience. They argue that language acquisition should be viewed as closely linked to social, emotional and cognitive domains, working memory systems, comprehension and production requirements, and the communicative contexts encountered. They rely on evidence from two atypical populations: Down Syndrome and Fragile-X Syndrome. In DS, the fractionation of language strengths and weakness is not what modularity would predict, falling out in terms of processing mode (comprehension vs. production), and distinguishing syntax from morphology. For FraX, in spite of the relative lack of detailed information that is currently available, the close association of language development with cognition and social experience challenges the autonomy of language.

3.5 Critical periods and implications for intervention

Lederberg and Spencer suggest that "research on the language of deaf people is uniquely well-suited to the study of critical periods" in language development. They make clear that we need to distinguish among different parts of the language system, not just levels such as syntax vs. vocabulary, but also in terms of processes, such as form vs. meaning mapping, speed of acquisition, etc. They provide a striking instance of cross-modal transfer in that late sign exposure may affect the development of phonological representation and or phonological processing, with lexical effects.

The theoretical consideration that emerges from early language exposure to either sign or spoken language is that the representation of language is not modality-specific. The clinical considerations that emanate from Schauwers et al. indicate that early cochlear implant fitting is desirable for the development of spoken language in deaf children. The important clinical implication from Mayberry's research (cited in Lederberg & Spencer this volume) is that early exposure to sign language does not impede the development of spoken language; in fact there appears to be an advantage for spoken language development in children who have been exposed to sign language at an early age.

HI is also the field with the single most striking intervention procedure – cochlear implantation (CI) (Schauwers et al.). Because this is a new treatment for deafness, the cochlear implant field is dominated by clinical studies where the main motivation for research is to assess the efficacy of the procedure. In clinical studies, research is conducted as part of ongoing clinical assessment and surveillance. Typically, the measures used are standardized assessments, for example, published assessments that have been normed on typically developing children, such as the Reynell Developmental Language Scales (Edwards, Fletcher, Hughes, Garman, Letts, & Sinka 1997) or standard assessment techniques such as profiling speech output according to voice, place and manner of articulation. Using measures such as these inevitably means that the research is dominated by a comparison of the outcomes of cochlear implant users against some sort of normative standard. In the main, the research is exploratory and descriptive. There is a clear clinical need to establish the efficacy of this new treatment for deaf children. On the basis of this type of research, clinicians can answer questions and make predictions about the likely rate and trajectory of speech and language development post cochlear implant fitting. This in turn means that expectations for language development can be based on evidence rather than opinion. Clinical research yields clinically valuable outcomes, but to what extent can these studies contribute to theoretical issues in language acquisition research? On the face of it, the opportunity to compare the language outcomes in deaf children relative to the timing of cochlear implant fitting is a fruitful way to explore the critical period hypothesis. The majority of cochlear implant studies that have investigated the impact of timing of cochlear implant fitting suggest that early intervention leads to better outcomes (Fryauf-Bertschy, Tyler, Kelsay, Gantz, & Woodworth 1997; O'Donoghue, Nikolopoulos, & Archbold 2000).

This conclusion, though, is as yet more clinically significant than theoretically valuable. There are several reasons for this. First, there is a lack of theoretically motivated studies where experimental rather than standard measures have been adopted. Secondly, as the age of implant fitting has reduced, candidacy criteria have also changed (i.e., children with less severe hearing impairment are now deemed suitable cochlear implant candidates). In addition, advances in cochlear implant technology have also occurred. Therefore, the comparison of timing of implant fit across cohorts, even when the same standard measures have been used, is potentially confounded by other factors. Thirdly, if we are to extract conclusions about critical periods from research that has compared children who received intervention early and those who received intervention later we would have to assume that, apart from the timing of intervention, the groups were the same in all other respects. Clinical experience suggests that this is not likely to be the case. In the UK at least, securing treatment quickly for children requires a high level of parental commitment and involvement. Given the impact that parent involvement seems to have on language outcomes in deaf children (see Moeller 2000, cited in Lederberg & Spencer in this volume), it is likely that children treated early also have highly involved parents. So, the degree of parental involvement rather than the age of treatment per se might be a causal factor in language outcomes following cochlear implant fitting.

4. Conclusions and directions for further research

Doing research with children from special populations is challenging: the clinical context constrains research design, testing methodologies, and sample size. In spite of these considerations, the contributions to this volume testify to the enormous progress that has been made over the last 20 years or so.

As already discussed in this volume (Abbeduto & Chapman; Thomas) the degree of variability within groups of children with developmental disorders is high (Karmiloff-Smith 1998; Pezzini, Vicari, Volterra, Milani, & Osssella 1999; Kjelgaard & Tager-Flusberg 2001; Stojanovik, Perkins, & Howard 2004). From a clinical perspective, it is of paramount importance for clinicians to be familiar with this variability in order to conduct appropriate assessments and plan intervention. From a theoretical perspective, if we continue to plan our research and analyze our data on the basis that we will find homogeneity within groups and heterogeneity between groups, then the combination of high variance in special populations and small sample sizes is potentially a very serious threat to the field's validity. Any manifestation of atypical language ability is a function of at least the following: the particular pattern or syndrome, the individual's own characteristic style, and the history of that individual to that point of development. We can start to ask whether this variance is a problem or whether the investigation of the source of variance can itself prove to be a fruitful area for research.

Regarding the patterns or syndromes, we have clear evidence in this volume of the complex nature of strengths and weakness within developmental profiles of particular disorders (Thomas; Abbeduto & Chapman); for example, research into SLI suggests different manifestations of the disorder, and several subgroups with strengths and weaknesses in different domains have been identified (Conti-Ramsden & Botting 1999). In relation to developmental variance, we have striking evidence in this volume of differential trajectories, and even of cross-over of the strands of relative strength and weakness over time (Thomas, Abbeduto, & Chapman). Accordingly, we endorse suggestions from a number of contributors that more longitudinal studies are required; we would also add that the single case-study paradigm advanced for aphasia research (Coltheart 1983) has potential for combining hypothetico-deductive investigation with treatment in ways that have yet to be tapped in research into childhood language impairment. Large-scale longitudinal studies also have an important role to play. But in each case, there must be a theoretically motivated starting point.

Advances in computational modeling, although in their infancy at present, have the potential to further our understanding of the constraints involved in typical language acquisition as well as optimizing the outcome of language learning in atypical populations. This raises the question, What are we looking for from special populations? One major issue that may be addressed is the relation between internal and external variables, including particularly the genotype-phenotype question. In this context, the type of language variation that can be exploited in cross-linguistic research may find a parallel in research with special populations. Perhaps a way forward would be to look for similar phenotypes across various genotypes in order to broaden our understanding of the gene-to-behavior mappings as well as to evaluate theoretical accounts of the organization of human cognition, in particular theories assuming the presence of innate modular structure. It may be that there is the need to move away from looking for dissociations of cognitive domains and pay more attention to the possible associations, which is what has been suggested by Abbeduto and Chapman as well as Thomas.

A further example may be found in the potential that research with deaf people has to provide an important perspective on language development and cognition. Emanating from Dodd's work on the phonological development of deaf children in the nineteen seventies (Dodd 1976), we now have a body of evidence which suggests that the acquisition of phonological knowledge and phonological representation in the mental lexicon is a-modal. Research has investigated the impact of the use of *cued speech* on phonological representation and phonological processing in deaf children and adults (Alegria, Leybaert, Charlier, & Hage 1992). Cued speech, devised by Cornett (1967), uses hand shape, hand movement and lip pattern in order to convey information to support speech perception. Experiments on short-term memory (Leybaert, Alegria, Hage, & Charlier 1998) and phonological awareness (Charlier & Leybaert 2000) show that deaf children and adults can develop phonological representations based on visual perception. Other research in the field of deafness shows that this flexibility in perceptual processing is not limited to the auditory and visual modalities. Short-term memory experiments show that deaf people who use finger-spelling exhibit the classic similarity effect when presented with lists of dactylically similar items to remember (Hanson, Liberman, & Shankweiler 1984). Taken together, these findings provide insight into both the *a-modal* nature of phonological representations and the *flexibility* of the development of mental representations. At an explanatory level, we might find support here for the theoretical position that phonological structure emerges as a result of the repeated exposure to the properties of the substance (Lindblom, MacNeilage, & Studdert-Kennedy 1984). It seems that phonological structure emerges regardless of the nature of the substance:

deaf people can derive phonological knowledge based on speech reading, cued speech, finger-spelling, sign language (Mayberry 1994) and spoken language (James, Rajput, Brown, Sirimana, Brinton, & Goswami in press; Kirk, Pisoni, & Osberger 1995). At the very least the current state of knowledge from deafness research should dispel any residual notion that phonology and speech are synonymous. What we might hope for is that research from deaf populations shapes future phonological theory. The richness that exists in modality amongst deaf populations provides a unique opportunity to explore the development of phonological knowledge at all three levels; perceptual, representational and motoric.

It seems clear from this review that our understanding of the centrality of phonology in the development of the lexicon is obscured because of a problem with definition. The term *phonology* is used in many studies when researchers are really referring to *speech* output. The set of terms that are used to describe the characteristic immaturities present in young children's speech or in the speech of children who have delayed speech development (e.g. phonological processes) have descriptive value, but it is not clear that these labels have explanatory power. In terms of clinical evaluation we assess phonology at three levels, input, representation and output. Deficits in input and representational phonology would lead to a clinical diagnosis of phonological impairment, but deficits in speech output might be due to articulation deficits and have no phonological basis. These articulatory impairments could still be described using phonological processes (e.g. gliding of liquids), but this description does not imply causation or provide any explanation. To elucidate this further, children with autism have been reported to have unusual sound substitutions or deletions in their speech output. Clinical experience with this population suggests that some high functioning verbal children who have autism do engage in systematic substitutions or additions of sounds. For example, children with otherwise intact speech production have been known to add a single consonant to the end or beginning of words (e.g., adding /g/ to the end of words), but they spontaneously cease this behavior or change the sound in favor of another one. Rather than viewing this type of behavior as a phonological delay or deficit, it seems more appropriate to interpret it in a way that is consistent with the underlying social-cognitive or cognitive impairment in autism. The sound substitutions and deletions could be viewed as a manifestation of the need for consistency, in this case the child is striving for consistency in speech production. As far as we are aware, there is no detailed research documentation of this phenomenon, but based on clinical experience we believe that this type of behavior is only found in high functioning children with autism who have developed spoken language. Exploring the interactions between the speech substitutions and lexical development in children with autism would undoubtedly be very interesting. We might predict that in this population there would be a positive correlation between speech substitutions and lexical development. However, the conclusions from such a study would be very different to those of a study which investigated these interactions in children in a population of children who had a core deficit in phonological representation. According to Metsala and Walley (1998), the expansion of the lexicon leads to segmental organization. If data from special populations can be used to inform mainstream theoretical debate, then we need to ensure that, (a) clinically motivated studies are based on up to date theoretical models, and (b) theoretically motivated studies are informed by clinical judgment.

References

Abbeduto, L. (Ed.). (2003). *International Review of Research in Mental Retardation, Volume 27: Language and Communication in Mental Retardation.* New York: Elsevier, Academic Press.

Abbeduto, L. (2004). "Communication challenges facing youth with fragile X syndrome." Presentation at the biennial international conference of the National Fragile X Foundation, Washington, DC.

Abbeduto, L. & Hagerman, R. (1997). "Language and communication in fragile X syndrome." *Mental Retardation and Developmental Disabilities Research Reviews, 3,* 313–322.

Abbeduto, L. & Murphy, M. M. (2004). "Language, social cognition, maladaptive behavior and communication in Down syndrome and fragile X syndrome." In M. Rice & S. F. Warren (Eds.), *Developmental Language Disorders: From phenotypes to etiologies* (pp. 77–97). Mahwah, NJ: Lawrence Erlbaum Associates.

Abbeduto, L., Evans, J., & Dolan, T. (2001a). "Theoretical perspectives on language and communication problems in mental retardation and developmental disabilities." *Mental Retardation and Developmental Disabilities Research Reviews, 7,* 45–55.

Abbeduto, L., Murphy, M. M., Cawthon, S. W., Richmond, E. K., Weissman, M. D., Karadottir, S., & O'Brien, A. (2003). "Receptive language skills of adolescents and young adults with down or fragile X syndrome." *American Journal on Mental Retardation, 108,* 149–160.

Abbeduto, L., Pavetto, M., Karadottir, S., O'Brien, A., Weissman, M., Kesin, E., & Cawthon, S. (2000). "Expressive language development in adolescents and young adults with fragile X syndrome: Relationships with nonverbal cognition and syndrome specificity." Paper presented at the 7th International Fragile X Conference, Los Angeles, CA.

Abbeduto, L., Pavetto, M., Kesin, E., Weissman, M., Karadottir, S., O'Brien, A., & Cawthon, S. (2001b). "The linguistic and cognitive profile of Down syndrome: Evidence from a comparison with fragile X syndrome." *Down Syndrome Research and Practice, 7,* 9–16.

Alegria, J., Leybaert, J., Charlier, B., & Hage, C. (1992). "On the origin of phonological representations in the deaf: Hearing lips and hands." In J. Alegria, D. Holender, J. Morais, J. Radeau, & M. Radeau (Eds.), *Analytic Approaches to Human Cognition* (pp. 107–132). Amsterdam: Elsevier.

Allen, D., Steinberg, M., Dunn, M., Fein, D., Feinstein, C., Waterhouse, L., & Rapin, I. (2001). "Autistic disorder versus other pervasive developmental disorders in young children: Same or different?" *European Journal of Child Adolescent Psychiatry, 10,* 67–78.

Allen, M. C., Nikolopoulos, T. P., & O'Donoghue, G. M. (1998). "Speech intelligibility in children after cochlear implantation." *The American Journal of Otology, 19*, 742–746.

Allen, S. E. & Dyar, D. (1997). "Profiling linguistic outcomes in young children after cochlear implantation." *The American Journal of Otology, 18*, 127–128.

American Psychiatric Association. (1994). *Diagnostic and Statistical Manual of Mental Disorders* (DSM-IV, 4th edition). Washington, DC: American Psychiatric Association.

Arehart, K. H., Yoshinaga-Itano, C., Thomson, V., Gabbard, S. A., & Stredler-Brown, A. (1998). "State of the states: The status of universal newborn hearing screening, assessment and intervention systems in 16 states." *American Journal of Audiology, 7*, 101–114.

Bailey, D. B., Bruer, J. T., Symons, F. J., & Lichtman, J. W. (Eds.). (2001). *Critical thinking about critical periods.* Baltimore, MD: Brookes.

Bailey, D. B., Jr., Hatton, D. D., & Skinner, M. (1998). "Early developmental trajectories of males with fragile X syndrome." *American Journal on Mental Retardation, 103*, 29–39.

Bailey, D. B., Jr., Hatton, D. D., Mesibov, G., & Ament, N. (2000b). "Early development, temperament and functional impairment in autism and fragile X syndrome." *Journal of Autism and Developmental Disorders, 30*, 49–59.

Bailey, D. B., Jr., Skinner, D., Hatton, D., & Roberts, J. (2000a). "Family experiences and factors associated with the diagnosis of fragile X syndrome." *Developmental and Behavioral Pediatrics, 21*, 315–321.

Baird, G., Cass, H., & Slonims, V. (2003). "Clinical review: Diagnosis of autism." *British Medical Journal, 327*, 488–493.

Baltaxe, C. & D'Angiola, N. (1996). "Referencing skills in children with autism and specific language impairment." *European Journal of Disorders of Communication, 31*, 245–258.

Baron-Cohen, S. & Staunton, R. (1994). "Do children with autism acquire the phonology of their peers? An examination of group identification through the window of bilingualism." *First Language, 14*, 241–248.

Bartak, L., Rutter, M., & Cox, A. (1975). "A comparative study of infantile autism and specific developmental receptive language disorder: I. The children." *British Journal of Psychiatry, 126*, 127–145.

Bartolucci, G., Pierce, S., & Streiner, D. (1980). "Cross-sectional studies of grammatical morphemes in autistic and mentally retarded children." *Journal of Autism and Developmental Disorders, 10*, 39–50.

Bates, E. (2004). "Explaining and interpreting deficits in language development across clinical groups: Where do we go from here?" *Brain and Language, 88*, 248–253.

Bates, E. & Goodman, J. (2001). "On the inseparability of grammar and the lexicon: Evidence from acquisition." In M. Tomasello & E. Bates (Eds.), *Language Development: The essential readings* (pp. 134–162). Malden, MA: Blackwell.

Bates, E. & Roe, K. (2001). "Language development in children with unilateral brain injury." In C. A. Nelson & M. Luciana (Eds.), *Handbook of Developmental Cognitive Neuroscience* (pp. 281–307). Cambridge, MA: The MIT Press.

Bauer, D., Goldfield, B., & Reznick, J. (2002). "Alternative approaches to analyzing individual differences in the rate of early vocabulary development." *Applied Psycholinguistics, 23*, 313–315.

Bauer, R. & Benedict, P. (1997). *Modern Cantonese Phonology.* Berlin: Mouton de Gruyter.

Baumgardner, T., Reiss, A. L., Freund, L., & Abrams M. T. (1995). "Specification of the neurobehavioral phenotype of males with fragile X syndrome." *Pediatrics, 95*, 744–752.

Behrend, D., Scofield, J., & Kleinknecht, E. (2001). "Beyond fast-mapping: Young children's extensions of novel words and novel facts." *Developmental Psychology, 37*, 698–705.

Belser, R. C. & Sudhalter, V. (1995). "Arousal difficulties in males with fragile X syndrome: A preliminary report." *Developmental Brain Dysfunction, 8*, 270–279.

Belser, R. C. & Sudhalter, V. (2001). "Conversational characteristics of children with fragile X syndrome: Repetitive speech." *American Journal on Mental Retardation, 106*, 28–38.

Bertrand, J., Mervis, C., Rice, C. E., & Adamson, L. (1993). "Development of joint attention by a toddler with Williams syndrome." Paper presented at the Gatlinberg Conference on Research and Theory in Mental Retardation and Developmental Disabilities, Gatlinberg.

Bishop, D. V. M. (1983). *The Test for Reception of Grammar.* Age and Cognitive Performance Research Centre, University of Manchester.

Bishop, D. V. M. (1989). "Autism, Asperger's syndrome and semantic-pragmatic disorder: Where are the boundaries?" *British Journal of Disorders of Communication, 24*, 107–121.

Bishop, D. V. M. (1997). "Cognitive neuropsychology and developmental disorders: Uncomfortable bedfellows." *Quarterly Journal of Experimental Psychology, 50A*, 899–923.

Bishop, D. V. M. (1999). "An innate basis for language?" *Science, 286*, 2283–2284.

Bishop, D. V. M. (2004). "Classification of developmental language disorders: Theoritical issues and clinical implications." In L. Verhoeven (Ed.), *Specific Language Impairment: Diagnostic dilemmas* (pp. 309–326). Mahwah, NJ: Lawrence Erlbaum Associates.

Bishop, D. V. M. & Norbury, C. (2002). "Exploring the borderlands of autistic disorder and specific language impairment: A study using standardized diagnostic instruments." *Journal of Child Psychology and Psychiatry, 37*, 391–403.

Blamey, P. J. (2003). "Development of spoken language by deaf children." In M. Marschark & P. E. Spencer (Eds.), *Oxford handbook of deaf studies, language and education* (pp. 232–246). NewYork: Oxford University Press.

Blamey, P. J., Barry, J. G., & Jacq, P. (2001). "Phonetic inventory development in young cochlear implant users 6 years postoperation." *Journal of Speech, Language and Hearing Research, 44*, 73–79.

Blanchard, J., Gangestad, S., Brown, S., & Horan, W. (2000). "Hedonic capacity and schizotypy revisited: A taxometric analysis of social anhedonia." *Journal of Abnormal Psychology, 109*, 87–95.

Bloom, L. (1970). *Language Development: Form and function in emerging grammars.* Cambridge, MA: The MIT Press.

Bloom, P. (2000). *How Children Learn the Meanings of Words.* Cambridge, MA: The MIT Press.

Bollard, P. M., Chute, P. M., Popp, A., & Parisier, S. C. (1999). "Specific language growth in young children using the Clarion cochlear implant." *Annals of Otology, Rhinology and Laryngology, 108*, 119–123.

Boothroyd, A. (1984). "Auditory perception of speech contrasts by subjects with sensorineural hearing loss." *Journal of Speech and Hearing Research, 27*, 134–144.

Boothroyd, A. & Boothroyd-Turner, D. (2002). "Postimplantation audition and educational attainment in children with prelingually acquired profound deafness." *Annals of Otology, Rhinology and Laryngology, 111*, 79–84.

Boothroyd, A., Geers, A. E., & Moog, J. S. (1991). "Practical implications of cochlear implants in children." *Ear and Hearing, 12*, 81–89.

Botting, N. & Conti-Ramsden, G. (2003). "Autism, primary pragmatic difficulties and specific language impairment: Can we distinguish them using psycholinguistic markers?" *Developmental Medicine and Child Neurology, 45*, 515–524.

Boudreau, D. & Chapman, R. S. (2000). "The relationship between event representation and linguistic skill in narratives of children and adolescents with Down syndrome." *Journal of Speech, Language and Hearing Research, 43*, 1146–1159.

Bregman, J. D., Leckman, J. F., & Ort, S. I. (1988). "Fragile X syndrome: Genetic predisposition to psychopathology." *Journal of Autism and Developmental Disorders, 18*, 343–354.

Brown, R. (1973). *A First Language: The early stages.* London: George Allen and Unwin.

Brown, W. T. (2002). "The molecular biology of the fragile X mutation." In R. J. Hagerman & P. J. Hagerman (Eds.), *Fragile X Syndrome: Diagnosis, treatment and research* (3rd edition, pp. 110–135). Baltimore, MD: Johns Hopkins University Press.

Bruer, J. T. (2001). "A critical and sensitive period primer." In D. B. Bailey, J. T. Bruer, F. J. Symons, & J. W. Lichtman (Eds.), *Critical Thinking about Crtical Periods* (pp. 3–26). Baltimore, MD: Brookes.

Bruner, J. S. (1983). *Child's Talk: Learning to use language.* Oxford: Oxford University Press.

Burack, J. A., Shulman, C., Katzir, E., Schaap, T., Brennan, J. M., Iarocci, G., Wilansky, P., & Amir, N. (1999). "Cognitive and behavioural development of Israeli males with fragile X and Down syndrome." *International Journal of Behavioral Development, 23*, 519–531.

Caplan, D. (1987). *Neurolinguistics and Linguistic Aphasiology.* Cambridge: Cambridge University Press.

Capone, N. C. & McGregor, K. K. (2004). "Gesture development: A review for clinical and review practices." *Journal of Speech, Language and Hearing Research, 47*, 173–186.

Carey, S. & Bartlett, E. (1978). "Acquiring a single new word." *Papers and Reports on Child Language Development, 15*, 17–29.

Chapman, R. S. (2000). "Children's language learning: An interactionist perspective." *Journal of Child Psychology and Psychiatry and Allied Disciplines, 41*, 33–54.

Chapman, R. S. (2003). "Language and communication in individuals with Down syndrome." In L. Abbeduto (Ed.), *International Review of Research in Mental Retardation: Language and communication, 27* (pp. 1–34). New York: Academic Press.

Chapman, R. S. & Hesketh, L. (2000). "The behavioral phenotype of Down syndrome." *Mental Retardation and Developmental Disabilities Research Review, 6*, 84–95.

Chapman, R. S., Kay-Raining Bird, E., & Schwartz, S. (1990). "Fast mapping of words in event contexts by children with Down syndrome." *Journal of Speech and Hearing Disorders, 55*, 761–770.

Chapman, R. S., Hesketh, L. J., & Kistler, D. (2002). "Predicting longitudinal change in language production and comprehension in individuals with Down syndrome: Hierarchical linear modeling." *Journal of Speech, Language and Hearing Research, 45*, 902–915.

Chapman, R. S., Schwartz, S. E., & Kay-Raining Bird, E. (1991). "Language skills of children and adolescents with Down syndrome I. Comprehension." *Journal of Speech and Hearing Research, 34*, 1106–1120.

Chapman, R. S., Seung, H.-K., Schwartz, S. E., & Kay-Raining Bird, E. (1998). "Language skills of children and adolescents with Down syndrome: II. Production deficits." *Journal of Speech, Language and Hearing Research, 41*, 861–873.

Chapman, R. S., Seung, H.-K., Schwartz, S. E., & Kay-Raining Bird, E. (2000). "Predicting language production in children and adolescents with Down syndrome: The role of comprehension." *Journal of Speech and Hearing Research, 43*, 340–350.

Charlier, B. & Leybaert, J. (2000). "The rhyming skills of deaf children educated with phonetically augmented speechreading." *Quarterly Journal of Experimental Psychology, 53A*(2), 349–375.

Charman, T., Drew, A., Baird, C., & Baird, G. (2003). "Measuring early language development in preschool children with autism spectrum disorder using the MacArthur Communicative Development Inventory (Infant Form)." *Journal of Child Language, 30*, 213–236.

Charman, T., Baron-Cohen, S., Swettenham, J., Baird, G., Drew, A., & Cox, A. (2003). "Predicting language outcome in infants with autism and pervasive developmental disorder." *International Journal of Language and Communication Disorders, 38*, 265–285.

Chiat, S. (2001). "Mapping theories of developmental language impairment: Premises, predictions and evidence." *Language and Cognitive Processes, 16*, 113–142.

Chiat, S. (2003). *Understanding Children with Language Problems.* Cambridge: Cambridge University Press.

Chin, S. B. (2002). "Aspects of stop consonant production by pediatric users of cochlear implants." *Language, Speech and Hearing Services in Schools, 33*, 38–51.

Chin, S. B. (2003). "Children's consonant inventories after extended cochlear implant use." *Journal of Speech, Language and Hearing Research, 46*, 849–862.

Chin, S. B. & Kaiser, C. L. (2000). "Measurement of articulation in pediatric users of cochlear implants." *The Volta Review, 102*(4), 145–156.

Chomsky, N. (1957). *Syntactic Structures.* The Hague: Mouton.

Chomsky, N. (1965). *Aspects of the Theory of Syntax.* Cambridge, MA: The MIT Press.

Christiansen, M. H. & Chater, N. (2001). *Connectionist Psycholinguistics.* Westport, CT: Ablex.

Clahsen, H. & Almazan, M. (1998). "Syntax and morphology in Williams Syndrome." *Cognition, 68*, 167–198.

Clahsen, H. & Temple, C. (2003). "Words and rules in Williams syndrome." To appear in Y. Levy & J. Schaeffer (Eds.), *Towards a Definition of Specific Language Impairment in Children* (pp. 323–353). Hillsdale, NJ: Lawrence Erlbaum Associates.

Clark, E. V. (2002). *First Language Acquisition.* Cambridge: Cambridge University Press.

Coerts, J. & Mills, A. (1994). "Spontaneous language development of young deaf children with a cochlear implant." *Annals of Otology, Rhinology and Laryngology, 166*, 385–387.

Coerts, J., Baker, A. E., van den Broek, P., & Brokx, J. (1996). "Language development by deaf children with cochlear implants." In C. E. Johnson & J. H. V. Gilbert (Eds.), *Children's language, 9* (pp. 219–234). Hillsdale, NJ: Lawrence Erlbaum Associates.

Cohen, I. L. (1995). "A theoretical analysis of the role of hyperarousal in the learning and behavior of fragile X males." *Mental Retardation and Developmental Disabilities Research Reviews, 1*, 286–291.

Cohen, I. L., Vietze, P. M., Sudhalter, V., Jenkins, E. C., & Brown, W. T. (1989). "Parent-child dyadic gaze patterns in fragile X males and in non-fragile X males with autistic disorder." *Journal of Child Psychology and Psychiatry, 30*, 845–856.

Coltheart, M. (1983). "Aphasia therapy research: A single-case study approach." In C. Code & D. J. Muller (Eds.), *Aphasia Therapy* (pp. 194–202). London: Arnold.

Connor, C. M. & Zwolan, T. A. (in press). "Examining multiple sources of influence on the reading comprehension of children who use cochlear implants." *Journal of Speech, Language and Hearing Research.*

Connor, C. M., Heiber, S., Arts, H. A., & Zwolan, T. A. (2000). "Speech, vocabulary and the education of children using cochlear implants: Oral or total communication?" *Journal of Speech, Language and Hearing Research, 43*, 1185–1204.

Connor, C. M., Raudenbush, S., Zwolan, T. A., Heavner, K., & Craig, H. (submitted). "Age at cochlear implantation effects on vocabulary growth: Indications of an early sensitive phase for language acquisition."

Conti-Ramsden, G. & Botting, N. (1999). "Classification of children with specific language impairment: Longitudinal classifications." *Journal of Speech, Language and Hearing Research, 42*, 1195–1204.

Cornett, O. (1967). "Cued speech." *American Annals of the Deaf, 112*, 3–13.

Cornish, K., Sudhalter, V., & Turk, J. (2004). "Attention and language in fragile X." *Mental Retardation and Developmental Disabilities Research Reviews, 10*, 11–16.

Crawford, D. C., Acuna, J. M., & Sherman, S. L. (2001). "FMR1 and the fragile X syndrome: Human genome epidemiology review." *Genetics in Medicine, 3*, 359–371.

Croft, W. (2001). *Radical Construction Grammar.* Oxford: Oxford University Press.

Cromer, R. (1994). "A case study of dissociations between language and cognition." In H. Tager-Flusberg (Ed.), *Constraints on Language Acquisition: Studies of atypical children* (pp. 141–153). Hillsdale, NJ: Lawrence Erlbaum Associates.

Crosson, J. & Geers, A. E. (2000). "Structural analysis of narratives produced by a group of young cochlear implant users." *Annals of Otology, Rhinology and Laryngology, 185*, 118–119.

Crosson, J. & Geers, A. E. (2001). "Analysis of narrative ability in children with cochlear implants." *Ear and Hearing, 22*, 381–394.

Crystal, D., Fletcher, P., & Garman, M. (1976). *The Grammatical Analysis of Language Disability.* London: Arnold.

Cullington, H., Hodges, A. V., Butts, S. L., Dolan-Ash, S., & Balkany, T. J. (2000). "Comparison of language ability in children with cochlear implants placed in oral and total communication educational settings." *Annals of Otology Rhinology and Laryngology, 185*, 121–123.

Cunningham, M. (1966). "A five-year study of the language of an autistic child." *Journal of Child Psychology and Psychiatry and Allied Disciplines, 7*, 143–154.

Cunningham, C. C., Glenn, S. M., Wilkinson, P., & Sloper, P. (1985). "Mental ability, symbolic play and receptive and expressive language of young children with Down's syndrome." *Journal of Child Psychology and Psychiatry and Allied Disciplines, 26*, 255–265.

Curtiss, S. (1977). *Genie: A psycholinguistic study of a modern-day "wild child."* New York: Academic Press.

Dawson, G., Webb, S., Schellenberg, G. D., Dager, S., Friedman, S., Aylward, E., & Richards, T. (2002). "Defining the broader phenotype of autism: Genetic, brain and behavioral perspectives." *Development and Psychopathology, 14*, 581–611.

Dawson, P. W., Blamey, P. J., Dettman, S. J., Barker, E. J., & Clark, G. M. (1995). "A clinical report on receptive vocabulary skills in cochlear implant users." *Ear and Hearing, 16*, 287–294.

Dawson, P. W., Blamey, P. J., Dettman, S. J., Rowland, L. C., Barker, E. J., Tobey, E. A., Busby, P. A., Cowan, R. C., & Clark, G. M. (1995). "A clinical report on speech production of cochlear implant users." *Ear and Hearing, 16*, 551–561.

de Villiers, P. & Pomerantz, S. B. (1992). "Hearing-impaired students learning new words from written context." *Applied Psycholinguistics, 13*, 409–431.

Demark, J. L., Feldman, M. A., & Holden, J. J. A. (2003). "Behavioral relationship between autism and fragile X syndrome." *American Journal of Medical Genetics, 108*, 314–326.

Dick, F., Bates, E., Wulfeck, B., Aydelott, J., Dronkers, N., & Gernsbacher, M. (2001). "Language deficits, localization and grammar: Evidence for a distributive model of language breakdown in aphasic patients and neurologically intact individuals." *Psychological Review, 108*(3), 759–788.

Dick, F., Wulfeck, B., Krupa-Kwiatkowski, M., & Bates, E. (2004). "The development of complex sentence interpretation in typically developing children compared with children with specific language impairments or early unilateral focal lesions." *Developmental Science, 7*(3), 360–377.

Dionne, G., Dale, P., Boivin, M., & Plomin, R. (2003). "Genetic evidence for bidirectional effects of early lexical and grammatical development." *Child Development, 74*, 394–412.

Dodd, B. (1976). "The phonological systems of deaf children." *Journal of Speech and Hearing Disorders, 41*, 185–198.

Dollaghan, C. (1987). "Fast mapping in normal and language-impaired children." *Journal of Speech and Hearing Disorders, 52*, 218–222.

Dollaghan, C. (in press). "Taxonometric analysis of specific language impairment in 3- and 4-year-old children." *Journal of Speech, Language and Hearing Research.*

Dollaghan, C. & Campbell, T. (1998). "Nonword repetition and child language impairment." *Journal of Speech, Language, and Hearing Research, 41*, 1136–1146.

Donnai, D. & Karmiloff-Smith, A. (2000) "Williams Syndrome: From genotype through to the cognitive phenotype." *American Journal of Medical Genetics, 97*, 164–171.

Dromi, E. (1999). "Early lexical development." In M. Barrett (Ed.), *The Development of Language* (pp. 99–129). Hove: Psychology Press.

Dunn, L., Dunn, L., Whetton, C., & Burley, J. (1997). *British Picture Vocabulary Scale-Revised.* Slough, Bucks: NFER-Nelson Publishing Company.

Dunn, L., Dunn, L., Whetton, C., & Pintillie, D. (1982). *British Picture Vocabulary Scale.* Slough, Bucks: NFER-Nelson Publishing Company.

Dunn, M., Flax, J., Slivinski, M., & Aram, D. (1996). "The use of spontaneous language measures as criteria for identifying children with specific language impairment: An attempt to reconcile clinical and research incongruence." *Journal of Speech and Hearing Research, 39*, 643–654.

Dyer-Friedman, J., Glaser, B., Hessl, D., Johnston, C., Huffman, L. C., Taylor, A., Wisbeck, J., & Reiss, A. L. (2002). "Genetic and environmental influences on the cognitive outcomes of children with fragile X syndrome." *Journal of the American Academy of Child and Adolescent Psychiatry, 41*, 237–244.

Dykens, E. M. & Kasari, C. (1997). "Maladaptive behavior in children with Prader-Willi syndrome, Down syndrome and nonspecific mental retardation." *American Journal of Mental Retardation, 102*, 228–237.

Dykens, E. M., Hodapp, R. M., & Evans, D. W. (1994). "Profiles and development of adaptive behavior in children with Down syndrome." *American Journal of Mental Retardation, 98*, 580–587.

Dykens, E. M., Hodapp, R. M., & Finucane, B. M. (2000). *Genetics and Mental Retardation Syndromes: A new look at behavior and interventions.* Baltimore, MD: Brookes.

Dykens, E. M., Hodapp, R. M., & Leckman, J. F. (1987). "Strengths and weaknesses in the intellectual functioning of males with fragile X syndrome." *American Journal on Mental Deficiency, 92*, 234–236.

Dykens, E. M., Hodapp, R. M., & Leckman, J. F. (1989). "Adaptive and maladaptive functioning of institutionalized and noninstitutionalized fragile X males." *Journal of the American Academy of Child and Adolescent Psychiatry, 26*, 427–430.

Dykens, E. M., Hodapp R. M., Ort, S. I., & Leckman, J. F. (1993). "Trajectory of adaptive behaviour in males with fragile X syndrome." *Journal of Autism and Developmental Disorders, 23*, 135–145.

Dykens, E. M., Hodapp, R. M., Ort, S., Finucane, B. M., Shapiro, L. R., & Leckman, J. F. (1989). "The trajectory of cognitive development in males with fragile X syndrome." *Journal of the American Academy of Child and Adolescent Psychiatry, 28*, 422–426.

Eadie, P. A., Fey, M. E., Douglas, J. M., & Parsons, C. L. (2002). "Profiles of grammatical morphology and sentence imitation in children with specific language impairment and Down syndrome." *Journal of Speech, Language and Hearing Research, 45*, 720–732.

Edwards, J. & Lahey, M. (1996). Auditory lexical decisions of children with specific language impairment. *Journal of Speech and Hearing Research, 39*, 1263–1273.

Edwards, S., Fletcher, P., Garman, M., Hughes, A., Letts, C., & Sinka, I. (1997). *The Reynell Developmental Language Scales III: University of Reading Edition.* Windsor: NFER-Nelson Publishing Company.

Eisenmajer, R. & Prior, M. (1991). "Cognitive linguistic correlates of "theory of mind" ability in autistic children". *British Journal of Developmental Psychology, 9*, 351–364.

Eisenmajer, R., Prior, M., Leekam, S., Wing, L., Ong, B., Gould, J., & Welham, M. (1998). "Delayed language onset as a predictor of clinical symptoms in pervasive developmental disorders." *Journal of Autism and Developmental Disorders, 28*, 527–533.

El-Hakim, H., Levasseur, J., Papsin, B. C., Panesar, J., Mount, R. J., Stevens, D., & Harrison, R. V. (2001). "Assessment of vocabulary development in children after cochlear implantation." *Archives of Otolaryngology, Head and Neck Surgery, 127*, 1053–1059.

Ellis Weismer, S. & Hesketh, L. (1996). "Lexical learning by children with specific language impairment: Effects of linguistic input presented at varying speaking rates." *Journal of Speech and Hearing Research, 39*, 177–190.

Ellis Weismer, S. & Hesketh, L. (1998). "The impact of emphatic stress in novel word learning by children with specific language impairment." *Journal of Speech, Language and Hearing Research, 41*, 1444–1458.

Elman, J. L., Bates, E. A., Johnson, M. H., Karmiloff-Smith, A., Parisi, D., & Plunkett, K. (1996). *Rethinking Innateness: A connectionist perspective on development.* Cambridge, MA: The MIT Press.

Emmorey, K. (2002). *Language, Cognition and the Brain.* Mahwah, NJ: Lawrence Erlbaum Associates.

Emmorey, K. & Corina, D. P. (1990). "Lexical recognition in sign language: Effects of phonetic structure and morphology." *Perceptual and Motor Skills, 71*, 1227–1252.

Emmorey, K., Bellugi, U., Friederici, A., & Horn, P. (1995). "Effects of age of acquisition on grammatical sensitivity: Evidence from on-line and off-line tasks." *Applied Psycholinguistics, 16*, 1–23.

Emmorey, K., Grant, R., & Ewan, B. (1994). "A new case of linguistic isolation: Preliminary report." Paper presented at the Boston University Conference on Language Development, Boston, MA.

Epstein, C. J., Korenberg, J. R., Anneren, G., Antonarakis, S. E., Ayme, S., Courchesne, E., Epstein, L. B., Fowler, A., Groner, Y., Huret, J. L., Kempter, T. L., Lott, I. T., Lubin, B. H., Magenis, E., Opitz, J. M., Patterson, D., Priest, J. H., Pueschel, S. M., Rapoport, S. I., Sinet, P. M., Tanzi, R. E., & de la Cruz, F. (1991). "Protocols to establish genotype-phenotype correlations in Down syndrome." *American Journal of Human Genetics, 49*, 207–235.

Ertmer, D. J. & Mellon, J. A. (2001). "Beginning to talk at 20 months: Early vocal development in a young cochlear implant recipient." *Journal of Speech, Language and Hearing Research, 44*, 192–206.

Ertmer, D. J., Kirk, K. I., Sehgal, S. T., Riley, A. I., & Osberger, M. J. (1997). "A comparison of vowel production by children with multichannel cochlear implants or tactile aids: Perceptual evidence." *Ear and Hearing, 18*, 307–315.

Ertmer, D. J., Strong, L. M., & Sadagopan, N. (2003). "Beginning to communicate after cochlear implantation: Oral language development in a young child." *Journal of Speech, Language and Hearing Research, 46*, 328–340.

Ertmer, D. J., Young, N., Grohne, K., Mellon, J. A., Johnson, C., Corbett, K., & Saindon, K. (2002). "Vocal development in young children with cochlear implants: Profiles and implications for intervention." *Language, Speech and Hearing Services in Schools, 33*, 184–195.

Eyer, J., Leonard, L., Bedore, L., McGregor, K., Anderson, B., & Viescas, R. (2002). "Fast mapping of verbs by children with specific language impairment." *Clinical Linguistics & Phonetics, 16*, 55–77.

Feinstein, C. & Reiss, A. L. (2001). "Autism: The point of view from fragile X studies." *Journal of Autism and Developmental Disorders, 28*, 393–405.

Fenson, L., Dale, P. S., Reznick, J. S., Bates, E., Thal, D. J., & Pethick, S. J. (1994). *Variability in Early Communicative Development. Monographs of the Society for Research in Child Development, 59*, 5, Serial No. 242.

Fenson, L., Dale, P. S., Resznick, S., Thal, D., Bates, E., Hartung, J., Pethick, S., & Reilly, J. S. (1993). *The MacArthur Communicative Development Inventories: User's guide and technical manual.* San Diego, CA: Singular.

Ferrier, L. J., Bashir, A. S., Meryash, D. L., Johnston, J., & Wolff, P. (1991). "Conversational skills of individuals with fragile X syndrome: A comparison with autism and Down syndrome." *Developmental Medicine and Child Neurology, 33*, 776–788.

Fey, M. & Proctor-Williams, K. (2000). "Recasting, elicited imitation and modelling in grammar intervention for children with specific language impairments." In D. V. M. Bishop & L. B. Leonard (Eds.), *Speech and Language Impairments in Children* (pp. 177–194). Hove: Psychology Press.

Filipek, P. A., Accardo, P. J., Baranek, G. T., Cook, Jr. E. H., Dawson, G., Gordon, B., Gravel, J. S., Johnson, C. P., Kellen, R. J., Levy, S. E., Minshew, N. J., Prizant, B. M., Rapin, I., Rogers, S. J., Stone, W. L., Teplin, S., Tuchman, R. F., & Volkmar, F. R. (1999). "The screening and diagnosis of autism spectrum disorders." *Journal of Autism and Developmental Disorders, 29*, 439–484.

Fisch, G. S., Holden, J. J. A., Carpenter, N. J., Howard-Peebles, P. N., Maddalena, A., Pandya, A., & Nance, W. (1999). "Age-related language characteristics of children and adolescents with fragile X syndrome." *American Journal of Medical Genetics, 83*, 253–256.

Fischer, S. D. (1998). "Critical periods for language acquisition: Consequences for deaf education." In A. Weisel (Ed.), *Issues Unresolved: New perspectives on language and deaf education* (pp. 9–26). Washington, DC: Gallaudet University Press.

Fletcher, P., Leonard, L., Wong, A. M.-Y., & Stokes, S. (in press). "The expression of aspect in Cantonese-speaking children with specific language impairment." *Journal of Speech and Hearing Research.*

Folstein, S. E., Santangelo, S. L., Gilman, S. E., Piven, J., Landa, R., Lainhart, J., Hein, J., & Wzorek, M. (1999). "Predictors of cognitive test patterns in autism families." *Journal of Child Psychology and Psychiatry, 40*, 1117–1128.

Fombonne, E., Bolton, P., Prior, J., Jordan, H., & Rutter, M. (1997). "A family study of autism: Cognitive patterns and levels in parents and siblings." *Journal of Child Psychology and Psychiatry, 38*, 667–683.

Fodor, J. (1983). *The Modularity of Mind.* Cambridge, MA: The MIT Press.

Forster, K. I. (1976). "Accessing the mental lexicon." In R. J. Wales & E. Walker (Eds.), *New Approaches to Language Mechanisms* (pp. 257–287). Amsterdam: North-Holland.

Fowler, A. (1998). "Language in mental retardation: Associations with and dissociations from general cognition." In J. A. Burack, R. M. Hodapp, & E. Zigler (Eds.), *Handbook of Mental Retardation and Development* (pp. 290–333). Cambridge: Cambridge University Press.

Fowler, A. E., Gelman, R., & Gleitman, L. R. (1994). "The course of language learning in children with Down syndrome." In H. Tager-Flusberg (Ed.), *Constraints on Language Acquisition* (pp. 91–140). Mahwah, NJ: Lawrence Erlbaum Associates.

Frawley, W. (2002). "Control and cross-domain mental computation: Evidence from language breakdown." *Computational Intelligence, 18*, 1–28.

Freund, L. S. & Reiss, A. L. (1991). "Cognitive profiles associated with the fra(X) syndrome in males and females." *American Journal of Medical Genetics, 38*, 542–547.

Freund, L. S., Reiss, A. L., & Abrams, M. T. (1993). "Psychiatric disorders associated with fragile X in the young female." *Pediatrics, 91*, 321–329.

Freund, L. S., Peebles, C. D., Aylward, E., & Reiss, A. L. (1995). "Preliminary report on cognitive and adaptive behaviours of preschool-aged males with fragile X." *Developmental Brain Dysfunction, 8*, 242–251.

Fryauf-Bertschy, H., Tyler, R. S., Kelsay, D. M., Gantz, B. J., & Woodworth, G. P. (1997). "Cochlear implant use by prelingually deafened children: The influences of age at implant and length of device use." *Journal of Speech Language and Hearing Research, 40*, 183–199.

Gardner, M. (1982). *Expressive One Word Picture Vocabulary Test (Upper Extension)*. Los Angeles, LA: Western Psychological Services.

Gathercole, S. & Baddeley, A. (1990). "Phonological memory deficits in language disordered children: Is there a causal connection?" *Journal of Memory and Language, 29*, 336–360.

Geers, A. E. (2002). "Factors affecting the development of speech, language and literacy in children with early cochlear implantation." *Language, Speech and Hearing Services in Schools, 33*, 172–183.

Geers, A. E. (in press). "Spoken language in children using cochlear implants." In P. E. Spencer & M. Marschark (Eds.), *Advances in Spoken Language Development of Deaf Children*. New York: Oxford University Press.

Geers, A. E. & Moog, J. (1994). "Spoken language results: Vocabulary, syntax and communication." *The Volta Review, 96*(5), 131–148.

Geers, A. E. & Tobey, E. A. (1992). "Effects of sensory aids on the development of speech production skills in children with profound hearing impairment." *The Volta Review, 94*, 135–163.

Geers, A. E., Brenner, C., Nicholas, J., Uchanski, R., Tye-Murray, N., & Tobey, E. A. (2002). "Rehabilitation factors contributing to implant benefit in children." *Annals of Otology, Rhinology and Laryngology, 111*, 127–130.

Gernsbacher, M., Sauer, E., Geye, H., O'Reilly, M., & Goldsmith, H. (submitted). "Early motor markers predict later speech within the autism spectrum."

Gillam, R. & Pearson, N. (2004). *Test of Narrative Language*. Austin, TX: PRO-ED.

Gilbertson, M. & Kamhi, A. G. (1995). "Novel word learning in children with hearing impairment." *Journal of Speech and Hearing Research, 38*, 630–642.

Gillis, S., Schauwers, K., & Govaerts, P. J. (2002). "Babbling milestones and beyond: Early speech development in CI children." In K. Schauwers, P. Govaerts, & S. Gillis (Eds.), *Antwerp Papers in Linguistics 102: Language acquisition in young children with a cochlear implant* (pp. 23–40). Antwerp: University of Antwerp.

Glaser, B., Hessl, D., Dyer-Friedman, J., Johnstone, C., Wisbeck, J., Taylor, A., & Reiss, A. (2003). "Biological and environmental contributions to adaptive behaviour in fragile X syndrome." *American Journal of Medical Genetics, 117A*, 21–29.

Gleitman, L. & Wanner, E. (1982). "Language acquisition: The state of the state of the art." In E. Wanner & L. Gleitman (Eds.), *Language Acquisition: The state of the art* (pp. 3–48). Cambridge: Cambridge University Press.

Gold, T. (1980). "Speech production in hearing-impaired children." *Journal of Communication Disorders, 13*, 397–418.

Goldberg, A. (1995). *Constructions: A construction grammar approach to argument structure.* Chicago, IL: University of Chicago Press.

Goldin-Meadow, S. (2002). "Getting a handle on language creation." In T. Givón & B. Malle (Eds.), *The Evolution of Language out of Pre-language* [Typological Studies in Language 53] (pp. 341–372). Amsterdam: John Benjamins.

Goldin-Meadow, S. (2003). *The Resilience of Language.* New York: Psychology Press.

Goldin-Meadow, S., Mylander, C., & Butcher, C. (1995). "The resilience of combinatorial structure at the word level: Morphology in self-styled gesture systems." *Cognition, 56*(3), 195–262.

Goldman, R. & Fristoe, M. (1986). *Goldman-Fristoe Test of Articulation.* Circle Pines, MN: American Guidance Service.

Golinkoff, R. M., Hirsh-Pasek, K., Bloom, L., Smith, L. B., Woodward, A. L., Akhtar, N., Tomasello, M., & Hollich, G. J. (2000). *Becoming a Word Learner: A debate on lexical acquisition.* New York: Oxford University Press.

Govaerts, P. J., De Beukelaer, C., Daemers, K., De Ceulaer, G., Yperman, M., Somers, T., Schatteman, I., & Offeciers, F. E. (2002). "Outcome of cochlear implantation at different ages from 0 to 6 years." *Otology and Neurotology, 23*, 885–890.

Greenough, W. T., Klintsova, A. Y., Irwin, S. A., Galvez, R., Bates, K. E., & Weiler, I. J. (2001). "Synaptic regulation of protein synthesis and the fragile X protein." *Proceedings of the National Academy of Sciences of the United States of America, 98*, 7101–7106.

Grela, B. G. (2003). "Do children with Down syndrome have difficulty with argument structure?" *Journal of Communication Disorders, 36*, 263–279.

Grice, S., Spratling, M. W., Karmiloff-Smith, A., Halit, H., Csibra, G., de Haan, M., & Johnson, M. H. (2001). "Disordered visual processing and oscillatory brain activity in autism and Williams syndrome." *Neuroreport, 12*, 2697–2700.

Griffith, P. L., Ripich, D. N., & Dastoli, S. L. (1990). "Narrative abilities in hearing-impaired children: Propositions and cohesion." *American Annals of the Deaf, 135*, 14–19.

Grimshaw, G. M., Adelstein, A., Bryden, M. P., & MacKinnon, G. E. (1998). "First-language acquisition in adolescence: Evidence for a critical period for verbal language development." *Brain and Language, 63*, 237–255.

Grogan, M. L., Barker, E. J., Dettman, S. J., & Blamey, P. J. (1995). "Phonetic and phonological changes in the connected speech of children using a cochlear implant." *Annals of Otology, Rhinology and Laryngology, 166*, 390–393.

Hagerman, R. J. (Ed.). (1999). *Neurodevelopmental Disorders.* Oxford: Oxford University Press.

Hagerman, R. J., Schreiner, R. A., Kemper, M. B., Wittenberger, M. D., Zahn, B., & Habicht, K. (1989). "Longitudinal IQ changes in fragile X males." *American Journal of Medical Genetics, 33*, 513–518.

Hammes, D. M., Novak, M. A., Rotz, L. A., Willis, M., Edmondson, D. M., & Thomas, J. F. (2002). "Early identification and cochlear implantation: Critical factors for spoken language development." *Annals of Otology, Rhinology and Laryngology, 111*, 74–78.

Hanson, V., Liberman, I., & Shankweiler, D. (1984). "Linguistic coding by deaf children in relation to beginning reading success." *Journal of Experimental Child Psychology, 37*, 378–393.

Happé, F. (1995). "The role of age and verbal ability in the theory of mind task performance of subjects with autism." *Child Development, 66*, 843–855.

Hart, B. & Risley, T. (1992). "American parenting of language-learning children: Persisting differences in family-child interactions observed in natural home environments." *Developmental Psychology, 28*(6), 1096–1105.

Hart, B. & Risley, T. (1995). *Meaningful Differences in Everyday Experiences of Young American Children.* Baltimore, MD: Brookes.

Hattori, M., Fujiyama, A., Taylor, T. D., Watanabe, H., Yada, T., Park, H. S., Toyoda, A., Ishii, K., Totoki, Y., Choi, D. K., Groner, Y., Soeda, E., Ohki, M., Takagi, T., Sakaki, Y., Taudien, S., Blechschmidt, K., Polley, A., Menzel, U., Delabar, J., Kumpf, K., Lehmann, R., Patterson, D., Reichwald, K., Rump, A., Schillhabel, M., Schudy, A., Zimmermann, W., Rosenthal, A., Kudoh, J., Schibuya, K., Kawasaki, K., Asakawa, S., Shintani, A., Sasaki, T., Nagamine, K., Mitsuyama, S., Antonarakis, S. E., Minoshima, S., Shimizu, N., Nordsiek, G., Hornischer, K., Brant, P., Scharfe, M., Schon, O., Desario, A., Reichelt, J., Kauer, G., Blocker, H., Ramser, J., Beck, A., Klages, S., Hennig S., Riesselmann, L., Dagand, E., Haaf, T., Wehrmeyer, S., Borzym, K., Gardiner, K., Nizetic, D., Francis, F., Lehrach, H., Reinhardt, R., Yaspo, M. L.; Chromosome 21 mapping and sequencing consortium. (2000). "The DNA sequence of human chromosome 21." *Nature, 405*, 311–319.

Heibeck, T. & Markman, E. (1987). "Word learning in children: An examination of fast mapping." *Child Development, 58*, 1021–1034.

Heilmann, J. (2004). *Research on specific language impairment: A review.* Working document, Language Analysis Lab. University of Wisconsin, Madison, WI.

Hesketh, L. J. & Chapman, R. S. (1998). "Verb use by individuals with Down syndrome." *American Journal on Mental Retardation, 103*, 288–304.

Higgins, M. B., Carney, A. E., McCleary, E., & Rogers, S. (1996). "Negative intraoral air pressures of deaf children with cochlear implants: Physiology, phonology and treatment." *Journal of Speech and Hearing Research, 39*, 957–967.

Hoff, E. & Naigles, L. (2002). "How children use input to acquire a lexicon." *Child Development, 73*, 418–433.

Howlin, P. (2003). "Outcome in high-functioning adults with autism with and without early language delays: Implications for the differentiation between autism and Asperger syndrome." *Journal of Autism and Developmental Disorders, 33*, 3–13.

Howlin, P., Mawhood, L., & Rutter, M. (2000). "Autism and developmental receptive language disorder – a follow-up comparison in early adult life. II: Social, behavioural and psychiatric outcomes." *Journal of Child Psychology and Psychiatry, 41*, 561–578.

Huttenlocher, J., Haight, W., & Bryk, A. (1991). "Early vocabulary growth: Relation to language input and gender." *Developmental Psychology, 27*(2), 236–248.

Huttenlocher, J., Vasilyeva, M., Cymerman, E., & Levine, S. (2002). "Language input and child syntax." *Cognitive Psychology, 45*(3), 337–374.

Iglesias, A. (2004). "Narrative language skills and reading achievement in bilingual children." Paper presented at the Symposium on Research in Child Language Development. University of Wisconsin, Madison, WI.

Illg, A., von der Haar-Heise, S., Goldring, J. E., Lesinski-Schiedat, A., Battmer, R. D., & Lenarz, T. (1999). "Speech perception results for children implanted with the Clarion cochlear implant at the medical university of Hannover." *Annals of Otology, Rhinology and Laryngology, 108*, 93–98.

Ingham, R., Fletcher, P., Schelletter, C., & Sinka, I. (1998). "Resultative VPs and specific language impairment." *Language Acquisition, 7*, 87–111.

Iverson, J. M., Longobardi, E., & Caselli, M. C. (2003). "Relationship between gestures and words in children with Down's syndrome and typically developing children in the early stages of communicative development." *International Journal of Language & Communication Disorders, 38*, 179–197.

Jackendoff, R. (2000). "Fodorian modularity and representational modularity." In Y. Grodzinsky, L. Shapiro, & D. Sweeney (Eds.), *Language and the Brain: Representation and processing* (pp. 3–30). San Diego, CA: Academic Press.

James, D., Rajput, K., Brown, T., Sirimana, T., Brinton, J., & Goswami, U. (in press). "Phonologial awareness in deaf children who use cochlear implants." *Journal of Speech Language and Hearing Research.*

Jaswal, V. & Markman, E. (2001). "Learning proper and common names in inferential versus obstensive contexts." *Child Development, 72*, 768–786.

Joanisse, M. F. & Seidenberg, M. S. (1999). "Impairments in verb morphology following brain injury: A connectionist model." *Proceedings of the National Academy of Science USA, 96*, 7592–7597.

Joanisse, M. F. & Seidenberg, M. S. (2003). "Phonology and syntax in specific language impairment: Evidence from connectionist model." *Brain and language, 86*, 40–56.

Johnston, J. (2004). "Fearless and bold in following ideas wherever they lead." The Elizabeth Bates Memorial Lecture, 25th Symposium on Research in Child Language Disorders, Madison, WI, June.

Johnston, J. & Schery, T. (1976). "The use of grammatical morphemes in children with communication disorders." In D. Morehead & M. Morehead (Eds.), *Normal and Deficient Child Language* (pp. 239–258). Baltimore, MD: University Park Press.

Jones, W., Bellugi, U., Lai, Z., Chiles, M., Reilly, J., Lincoln, A., & Adolphs, R. (2000). "Hypersociability in Williams syndrome." *Journal of Cognitive Neuroscience, 12*, (supplement), 30–46.

Joseph, R., Tager-Flusberg, H., & Lord, C. (2002). "Cognitive profiles and social-communicative functioning in children with autism." *Journal of Child Psychology and Psychiatry, 43*, 807–821.

Kanner, L. (1985). "Autistic disturbances of affective contact." In A. M. Donnellan (Ed.), *Classic readings in autism* (pp. 11–52). New York: Teachers College Press.

Karmiloff-Smith, A. (1997). "Crucial differences between developmental cognitive neuroscience and adult neuropsychology." *Developmental Neuropsychology, 13*(4), 513–524.

Karmiloff-Smith, A. (1998). "Development itself is the key to understanding developmental disorders." *Trends in Cognitive Sciences, 2*(10), 389–398.

Karmiloff-Smith, A. & Thomas, M. S. C. (2003). "What can developmental disorders tell us about the neurocomputational constraints that shape development? The case of Williams syndrome." *Development and Psychopathology, 15*, 969–990.

Karmiloff-Smith, A., Grant, J., Berthoud, I., Davies, M., Howlin, P., & Udwin, O. (1997). "Language and Williams syndrome: How intact is 'intact'?" *Child Development, 68*, 246–262.

Karmiloff-Smith, A., Thomas, M. S. C., Annaz, D., Humphreys, K., Ewing, S., Grice, S., Brace, N., Van Duuren, M., Pike, G., & Campbell, R. (2004). "Exploring the Williams Syndrome face processing debate: The importance of building developmental trajectories." *Journal of Child Psychology and Psychiatry and Allied Disciplines, 45*(7), 1258–1274.

Karmiloff-Smith, A., Tyler, L. K., Voice, K., Sims, K., Udwin, O., Howlins, P., & Davies, M. (1998). "Linguistic dissociations in Williams syndrome: evaluating receptive syntax in on-line and off-line tasks." *Neuropsychologia, 36*, 343–351.

Kasari, C., Freeman, S., Mundy, P., & Sigman, M. (1995). "Attention regulation by children with Down syndrome: Coordinated joint attention and social referencing looks." *American Journal on Mental Retardation, 100*, 128–136.

Kasari, C., Freeman, S. F., & Bass, W. (2003). "Empathy and response to distress in children with Down syndrome." *Journal of Child Psychology and Psychiatry, 44*, 424–431.

Kasari, C., Freeman, S. F., & Hughes, M. A. (2001). "Emotion recognition by children with Down syndrome." *American Journal of Mental Retardation, 106*, 59–72.

Kasari, C., Sigman, M., Mundy, P., & Yirmiya, N. (1990). "Affective sharing in the context of joint attention interactions of normal, autistic and mentally retarded children." *Journal of Autism and Developmental Disorders, 20*, 87–100.

Kegl, J., Senghas, A., & Coppola, M. (1999). "Creation through contact: Sign language emergence and sign language change in Nicaragua." In M. DeGraff (Ed.), *Language Creation and Language Change* (pp. 179–237). Cambridge, MA: The MIT Press.

King, C. & Quigley, S. P. (1985). *Reading and deafness.* Austin: PRO-ED.

Kirk, K. I. & Hill-Brown, C. (1985). "Speech and language results in children with a cochlear implant." *Ear and Hearing, 6*(3), 36–47.

Kirk, K. I., Diefendorf, E., Riley, A., & Osberger, M. J. (1995). "Consonant production by children with multichannel cochlear implants or hearing aids." *Advances in Otorhinolaryngology, 50*, 154–159.

Kirk, K. I., Miyamoto, R. T., Lento, C. L., Ying, E., O'Neill, T., & Fears, B. (2002). "Effects of age at implementation in young children." *Annals of Otology, Rhinology and Laryngology, 111*, 69–78.

Kirk, K. I., Miyamoto, R. T., Ying, E. A., Perdew, A. E., & Zuganelis, H. (2000). "Cochlear implantation in young children: Effects of age at implantation and communication mode." *The Volta Review, 102*(4), 127–144.

Kirk, K. I., Pisoni, D. B., & Osberger, M. J. (1995). "Lexical effects on spoken word recognition by pediatric cochlear implant users." *Ear and Hearing, 16*(5), 470–481.

Kishon-Rabin, L., Taitelbaum, R., Muchnik, C., Gehtler, I., Kronenberg, J., & Hildesheimer, M. (2002). "Development of speech perception and production in children with cochlear implants." *Annals of Otology, Rhinology and Laryngology, 111*, 85–90.

Kjelgaard, M. & Tager-Flusberg, H. (2001). "An investigation of language impairment in autism: Implications for genetic subgroups." *Language and Cognitive Processes, 16*, 287–308.

Klecan-Aker, J. & Blondeau, R. (1990). "An examination of written stories of hearing-impaired school-age children." *The Volta Review, 92*, 275–282.

Klee, T. (1992). "Developmental and diagnostic characteristics of quantitative measures of children's language production." *Topics in Language Disorders, 12*, 28–41.

Klee, T., Stokes, S., Wong, A., Fletcher, P., & Gavin, W. (2004). "Utterance length and lexical diversity in Cantonese-speaking children with and without language impairment." *Journal of Speech, Language and Hearing Research, 47*, 1396–1410.

Korenberg, J. R., Chen, X.-N., Schipper, R., Sun, Z., Gonsky, R., Gerwehr, S., Carpenter, N., Daumer, C., Dignan, P., Disteche, C., Graham, J. M., Jr., Hugdins, L., McGillivray, B., Miyazaki, K., Ogasawara, N., Park, J. P., Pagon, R., Pueschel, S., Sack, G., Say, B., Schuffenhauer, S., Soukup, S., & Yamanaka, T. (1994). "Down syndrome phenotypes: The consequences of chromosomal imbalance." *Proceedings of the National Academy of Science USA, 91*, 4997–5001.

Kuhl, P. K. (2000). "A new view of language acquisition." *PNAS, 97*, 11850–11857.

Kumin, L. (1994). "Intelligibility of speech in children with Down syndrome in natural settings: Parents' perspectives." *Perception and Motor Skills, 78*, 307–313.

Kuo, S. C. L. & Gibson, W. P. R. (2000). "The influence of residual high-frequency hearing on the outcome in congenitally deaf cochlear implant recipients." *The American Journal of Otology, 21*, 657–662.

Laing, E., Butterworth, G., Ansari, D., Gsödl, M., Laing, E., Barnham, Z., Lakusta, L., Tyler, L. K., Grice, S., Paterson, S., & Karmiloff-Smith, A. (2002). "Atypical linguistic and socio-communicative development in toddlers with Williams syndrome." *Developmental Science, 5*(2), 233–246.

Lavric, A., Pizzagalli, D., Forstmeier, S., & Rippon, G. (2001). "Mapping dissociations in verb morphology." *Trends in Cognitive Sciences, 5*, 301–308.

Laws, G. & Gunn, D. (2004). "Phonological memory as a predictor of language comprehension in Down syndrome: A five-year follow-up study." *Journal of Child Psychology and Psychiatry, 45*, 326–337.

Lederberg, A. R. & Everhart, V. S. (1998). "Communication between deaf children and their hearing mothers: The role of language, gesture and vocalizations." *Journal of Speech, Language and Hearing Research, 41*, 887–899.

Lederberg, A. R. & Spencer, P. E. (2001). "Vocabulary development of deaf and hard of hearing children." In M. D. Clark, M. Marschark, & M. Karchmer (Eds.), *Context, Cognition and Deafness* (pp. 88–112). Washington, DC: Gallaudet University Press.

Lederberg, A. R., Prezbindowski, A. K., & Spencer, P. E. (2000). "Word learning skills of deaf preschoolers: The development of novel mapping and rapid word learning strategies." *Child Development, 53*, 1055–1065.

Lederberg, A. R., Spencer, P. E., & Huston, S. (2003). "Development of fast-mapping in deaf and hard of hearing children: A longitudinal study." Paper presented at the Society for Research in Child Development, Tampa, FL.

Lee, T. H.-T., Wong, C. H., & Wong, C. S.-P. (1996). "Functional categories in child Cantonese." In T. H.-T. Lee, C. H. Wong, C. S. Leung, P. Man, A. Cheung, K. Szeto, & C. S.-P. Wong (Eds.), *The Development of Grammatical Competence in Cantonese-speaking Children* (pp. 1991–1994). Report of Hong Kong RGC Ear-marked grant.

Lenarz, T., Lesinski-Schiedat, A., von der Haar-Heise, S., Illg, A., Bertram, B., & Battmer, R. D. (1999). "Cochlear implantation in children under the age of two: The MHH experience with the Clarion cochlear implant." *Annals of Otology, Rhinology and Laryngology, 108*, 44–49.

Lenneberg, E. H. (1967). *Biological Foundations of Language*. New York: Wiley.

Leonard, L. B. (1983). "Discussion: Part II: Defining the boundaries of language disorders in children." In J. Miller, D. Yoder, & R. Schiefelbusch (Eds.), *Contemporary Issues in Language Intervention* [ASHA Reports 12] (pp. 107–112). Rockville, MD: The American Speech-Language-Hearing Association.

Leonard, L. (1992). "The use of morphology by children with specific language impairment: Evidence from three languages." In R. S. Chapman (Ed.), *Processes in Language Acquisition and Disorders* (pp. 186–201). St. Louis, MS: Mosby Year Book.

Leonard, L. B. (1998). *Children with Specific Language Impairment*. Cambridge, MA: The MIT Press.

Leonard, L. B. (2000). "SLI across languages." In D. V. M. Bishop & L. B. Leonard (Eds.), *Speech and Language Impairments in Children: Causes, characteristics, intervention and outcome* (pp. 115–129). Hove: Psychology Press.

Leonard, L. B. & Deevy, P. (2004). "Lexical deficits in specific language impairment." In L. Verhoeven & H. van Balkom (Eds.), *Classification of Developmental Language Disorders: theoretical issues and clinical implications* (pp. 209–233). Mahwah, NJ: Lawrence Erlbaum Associates.

Leung, C. S. (1995). The Development of Aspect Markers in a Cantonese-speaking Child between the Ages of 21 and 45 Months. Unpublished Ph.D. dissertation, University of Hawaii.

Levin, B. (1993). *English Verb Classes and Alternations: A preliminary investigation*. Chicago, IL: Chicago University Press.

Leybaert, J. & D'Hondt, M. (2003). "Neurolinguistic development in deaf children: The effect of early language experience." *International Journal of Audiology, 42*, Suppl. 1, 34–40.

Leybaert, J., Alegria, J., Hage, C., & Charlier, B. (1998). "The effect of exposure to phonetically augmented lipspeech in the prelingual deaf." In R. Campbell, B. Dodd, & D. Burnham (Eds.), *Hearing by Eye II* (pp. 283–302). Hove: Psychology Press.

Lindblom, B., MacNeilage, P., & Studdert-Kennedy, M. (1984). "Self-organizing processes and the explanation of phonological universals." In B. Butterworth, B. Comrie, & O. Dahl (Eds.), *Explanations for Language Universals* (pp. 181–203). New York: Mouton.

Linguistic Society of Hong Kong. (1974). *The LSHK Cantonese Romanization Scheme*. Hong Kong: Linguistic Society of Hong Kong.

Lord, C., Rutter, M., Goode, S., Heemsbergen, J., Jordan, H., Mawhood, L., & Schopler, E. (1989). "Autism diagnostic observation schedule: A standardized observation of communicative and social behavior." *Journal of Autism and Developmental Disorders, 19*, 185–212.

Loveland, K. A. & Landry, S. H. (1986). "Joint attention and language in autism and developmental language delay." *Journal of Autism and Developmental Disorders, 16*, 335–349.

Lutman, M. E. & Tait, D. M. (1995). "Early communicative behavior in young children receiving cochlear implants: Factor analysis of turn-taking and gaze orientation." *Annals of Otology, Rhinology and Laryngology, 166*, 397–399.

MacWhinney, B. (Ed.). (1999). *The Emergence of Language.* Mahwah, NJ: Lawrence Erlbaum Associates.

Madison, L. S., George, C., & Moeschler, J. B. (1986). "Cognitive functioning in the fragile X syndrome: A study of intellectual, memory and communication skills." *Journal of Mental Deficiency Research, 30*, 129–148.

Maitel, S., Dromi, E., Sagi, A., & Bornstein, M. (2000). "The Hebrew communicative development inventory: Language specific properties and cross-linguistic generalizations." *Journal of Child Language, 27*, 43–67.

Majerus, S. (2004). "Phonological processing in Williams syndrome." In S. Bartke & J. Siegmuller (Eds.), *Williams Syndrome: A cross-linguistic approach* (pp. 125–142). Amsterdam: John Benjamins.

Majerus, S., Palmisano, I., van der Linden, M., Barisnikov, K., & Poncelet, M. (2001). "An investigation of phonological processing in Williams syndrome." *Journal of the International Society, 7*(2), 153.

Malvern, D., Richards, B., Chipere, N., & Duran, P. (2004). *Lexical Diversity and Language Development.* Basingstoke: Palgrave.

Marcell, M. M. & Weeks, S. L. (1988). "Short-term memory difficulties in Down's syndrome." *Journal of Mental Deficiency Research, 32*, 153–162.

Marchman, V. & Bates, E. (1994). "Continuity in lexical and morphological development: A test of the critical mass hypothesis." *Journal of Child Language, 21*, 339–366.

Mareschal, D., Johnson, M., Sirios, S., Spratling, M., Thomas, M. S. C., & Westermann, G. (forthcoming). *Neuroconstructivism: How the brain constructs cognition.* Oxford: Oxford University Press.

Markson, L. & Bloom, P. (2001). "Evidence against a dedicated system for word learning in children." *Nature, 385*, 813–815.

Marschark, M., Mouradian, R., & Halas, M. (1994). "Discourse rules in the language productions of deaf and hearing children." *Journal of Experimental Child Psychology, 57*, 89–107.

Marshall, (1984). "Multiple perspectives on modularity." *Cognition, 17*, 209–242.

Masataka, N. (2000). "Information from speech and gesture is integrated when meanings of new words are categorized in normal young children but not in children with Williams syndrome." *Bulletin of the Japanese Cognitive Science Society, 7*, 37–51.

Masataka, N. (2001). "Why early linguistic milestones are delayed in children with Williams syndrome: late onset of hand banging as a possible rate-limiting constraint on the emergence of canonical babbling." *Developmental Science, 4*, 158–164.

Matthews, S. & Yip, V. (1994). *Cantonese: A comprehensive grammar.* London: Routledge.

Mayberry, R. I. (1993). First language acquisition after childhood differs from second language acquisition: The case of American Sign Language." *Journal of Speech and Hearing Research, 36*, 1258–1270.

Mayberry, R. I. (1994). "The importance of childhood to language acquisition: Evidence from American Sign Language." In J. C. Goodman & H. C. Nusbaum (Eds.), *The Development of Speech Perception: The transition from speech sounds to spoken words* (pp. 58–90). London: The MIT Press.

Mayberry, R. I. & Eichen, E. B. (1991). "The long-lasting advantage of learning sign language in childhood: Another look at the critical period for language acquisition." *Journal of Memory and Language, 30*, 486–512.

Mayberry, R. I. & Fischer, S. D. (1989). "Looking through phonological shape to lexical meaning: The bottleneck of non-native sign language processing." *Memory and Cognition, 17*(6), 740–753.

Mayberry, R. I. & Lock, E. (2003). "Age constraints in first versus second language acquisition: Evidence for linguistic plasticity and epigensis." *Brain and Language, 87*, 369–384.

Mayberry, R. I. & Witcher, P. E. (2002). "Native and non-native phonology effects on lexical access in ASL." Paper presented at the 43rd Annual Meeting of the Psychonomic Society, Kansas City, KS.

Mayes, S. D. & Calhoun, S. L. (2001). "Non-significance of early speech delay in children with autism and normal intelligence and implications for DSM-IV Asperger's disorder." *Autism, 5*, 81–94.

Mayne, A. M., Yoshinaga-Itano, C., Sedey, A. L., & Carey, A. (2000a). "Expressive vocabulary development of infants and toddlers who are deaf or hard of hearing." *The Volta Review, 100*(5), 1–28.

Mayne, A. M., Yoshinaga-Itano, C., Sedey, A. L., & Carey, A. (2000b). "Expressive vocabulary development of infants and toddlers who are deaf or hard of hearing." *The Volta Review, 100*(5), 29–52.

Mazzocco, M. M. M. (2000). "Advances in research on the fragile X syndrome." *Mental Retardation and Developmental Disabilities Research Reviews, 6*, 96–106.

Mazzocco, M. M. M., Pennington, B., & Hagerman, R. J. (1993). "The neurocognitive phenotype of female carriers of fragile X: Further evidence for specificity." *Journal of Development and Behavioral Pediatrics, 14*, 328–335.

McArthur, G. M. & Bishop, D. V. M. (2004). "Which people with specific language impairment have auditory processing deficits?" *Cognitive Neuropsychology, 21*, 79–94.

McCaffrey, H. A., Davis, B., MacNeilage, P. F., & von Hapsburg, D. (1999). "Multichannel cochlear implantation and the organization of early speech." *The Volta Review, 101*(1), 5–29.

McCann, J. & Peppé, S. (2003). "Prosody in autism spectrum disorders: A critical review." *International Journal of Language and Communication Disorders, 38*, 325–350.

McLean, L. & Cripe, J. (1997). "The effectiveness of early intervention for children with communication disorders." In M. J. Guralnick (Ed.), *The Effectiveness of Early Intervention.* Baltimore, MD: Brookes.

McLean, J., Yoder, D., & Schiefelbusch, R. (Eds.). (1972). *Language Intervention with the Retarded: Developing strategies.* Baltimore, MD: University Park Press.

McDonald, J. L. (1997). "Language acquisition: The acquisition of linguistic structure in normal and special populations." *Annual Review of Psychology, 48,* 215–241.

McGarr, N. S. (1983). "The intelligibility of deaf speech to experienced and inexperienced listeners." *Journal of Speech and Hearing Research, 26,* 451–458.

Meadow-Orlans, K. P., Spencer, P. E., & Koester, L. S. (in press). *The World of the Deaf Infant: A longitudinal study.* New York: Oxford University Press.

Mervis, C. B. & Bertrand, J. (1997). "Developmental relations between cognition and language: Evidence from Williams syndrome." In L. B. Adamson & M. A. Romski (Eds.), *Research on Communication and Language Disorders: Contributions to theories of language development* (pp. 75–106). Baltimore, MD: Brookes.

Mervis, C. B. & Robinson, B. F. (2000). "Expressive vocabulary of toddlers with Williams syndrome or Down syndrome: A Comparison." *Developmental Neuropsychology, 17,* 111–126.

Mervis, C. B., Morris, C. A., Bertrand, J., & Robinson, B. F. (1999). "William syndrome: Findings from an integrated program of research." In H. Tager-Flusberg (Ed.), *Neurodevelopmental Disorders: Contributions to a new framework from the cognitive neurosciences* (pp. 65–110). Cambridge, MA: The MIT Press.

Metsala, J. L. & Walley, A. C. (1998). "Spoken vocabulary growth and the segmental restructuring of lexical representations: Precursors to phonemic awareness and early reading ability." In J. L. Metsala & L. C. Ehri (Eds.), *Word Recognition in Beginning Literacy* (pp. 89–120). Hillsdale, NJ: Lawrence Erlbaum Associates.

Miles, S. & Chapman, R. S. (2002). "Narrative content as described by individuals with Down syndrome and typically developing children." *Journal of Speech, Language and Hearing Research, 45,* 175–189.

Miller, J. F. (1981). *Assessing Language Production in Children: Experimental procedures.* Baltimore, MD: University Park Press.

Miller, J. F. (1983). "Identifying children with language disorders and describing their language performance." In J. Miller, D. Yoder, & R. Schiefelbusch (Eds.), *Contemporary Issues in Language Intervention* [ASHA Reports 12] (pp. 61–74). Rockville, MD: The American Speech-Language-Hearing Association.

Miller, J. F. (1991). "Quantifying productive language disorders." In J. F. Miller (Ed.), *Research on Child Language Disorders: A decade of progress* (pp. 211–220). Austin, TX: Pro-Ed.

Miller, J. F. (1995). "Individual differences in vocabulary acquisition in children with Down syndrome." *Progress in Clinical Biology Research, 393,* 93–103.

Miller, J. F. (1999). "Profiles of language development in children with Down syndrome." In J. F. Miller, M. Leddy, & L. A. Leavitt (Eds.), *Improving the Communication of People with Down Dyndrome* (pp. 11–40). Baltimore, MD: Brookes.

Miller, J., Lall, V., Hollar, C., Jones, M., Lodholtz, C., Pech, S., Rolland, M., Tarnow, M., Vernon, M., Wood, M., & Dagget, B. (2001). "*Documenting age-related changes in language production.*" Presented at the Annual convention of the American Speech-Language-Hearing Association, New Orleans, LA.

Miller, J. F. & Ozonoff, S. (1997). "Did Asperger's cases have Asperger disorder? A research note." *Journal of Child Psychology and Psychiatry, 38*, 247–251.

Miller, J. & Yoder, D. (1972). "A Syntax Teaching Program." In J. McLean, D. Yoder, & R. Schiefelbush (Eds.), *Language Intervention with the Retarded: Developing strategies.* Baltimore, MD: University Park Press.

Miller, J. & Yoder, D. (1974). "An ontogenetic language teaching strategy for retarded children." In R. Schiefelbusch & L. Lloyd (Eds.), *Language Perspectives-Acquisition, Retardation and Intervention.* Baltimore, MD: University Park Press.

Mills, D. L., Alvarez, T. D., St. George, M., Appelbaum, L. G., Bellugi, U., & Neville, H. (2000). "Electrophysiological studies of face processing in Williams syndrome." *Journal of Cognitive Neuroscience, 12*, 47–64.

Mirrett, P. L., Bailey, D. B., Jr., Roberts, J. E., & Hatton, D. D. (2004). "Developmental screening and detection of developmental delays in infants and toddlers with fragile X syndrome." *Journal of Developmental and Behavioral Pediatrics, 25*, 21–27.

Mirrett, P. L., Roberts, J. E., & Price, J. (2003). "Early intervention practices and communication intervention strategies for young males with fragile X syndrome." *Language, Speech and Hearing Services in Schools, 34*, 320–331.

Miyamoto, R. T., Kirk, K. I., Svirsky, M. A., & Sehgal, S. T. (1999). "Communication skills in pediatric cochlear implant recipients." *Acta Otolaryngolica, 119*, 219–224. Stockholm.

Miyamoto, R. T., Svirsky, M. A., & Robbins, A. M. (1997). "Enhancement of expressive language in prelingually deaf children with cochlear implants." *Acta Otolaryngolica* (Stockholm), *117*, 154–157.

Moeller, M. P. (2000). "Early intervention and language development in children who are deaf and hard of hearing." *Pediatrics, 106*(3), e43, 41–49.

Moeller, M. P., Osberger, M. J., & Eccarius, M. (1986). "Receptive language skills." *Language and learning skills in hearing-impaired children, 23*, 41–53.

Mondain, M., Sillon, M., Vieu, A., Lanvin, M., Reuillard-Artieres, F., Tobey, E. A., & Uziel, A. (1997). "Speech perception skills and speech production intelligibility in French children with prelingual deafness and cochlear implants." *Archives of Otolaryngology, Head and Neck Surgery, 123*, 181–184.

Monsen, R. B. (1978). "Toward measuring how well hearing-impaired children speak." *Journal of Speech and Hearing Research, 21*, 197–219.

Monsen, R. B. (1983). "The oral speech intelligibility of hearing-impaired talkers." *Journal of Speech and Hearing Disorders, 48*, 286–296.

Moog, J. S. (2002). "Changing expectations for children with cochlear implants." *Annals of Otology, Rhinology and Laryngology, 111*, 138–142.

Moog, J. S. & Geers, A. E. (1999). "Speech and language acquisition in young children after cochlear implantation." *Otolaryngologic Clinics of North America, 32*(6), 1127–1141.

Moore, J. A. & Bass-Ringdahl, S. (2002). "Role of infant vocal development in candidacy for and efficacy of cochlear implantation." *Annals of Otology, Rhinology and Laryngology, 111*, 52–55.

Morehead, D. M. & Ingram, D. (1976). "The development of base syntax in normal and linguistically deviant children." In D. Morehead & M. Morehead (Eds.), *Normal and Deficient Child Language* (pp. 209–238). Baltimore, MD: The University Park Press.

Morehead, D. M. & Morehead, A. E. (Eds.). (1976). *Normal and Deficient Child Language.* Baltimore, MD: University Park Press.

Morford, J. P. (1996). "Insights to language from the study of gesture: A review of research on the gestural communication of non-signing deaf people." *Language and Communication, 16*(2), 165–178.

Morford, J. P. (1998). "Gesture when there is no speech model." *New Directions for Child Development, 79,* 101–106.

Morford, J. P. (2003). "Grammatical development in adolescent first-language learners." *Linguistics, 41,* 681–721.

Morford, J. P. & Goldin-Meadow, S. (1997). "From here and now to there and then: The development of displaced reference in homesign and English." *Child Development, 68*(3), 420–435.

Morford, J. P., Singleton, J. L., & Goldin-Meadow, S. (1995a). "From homesign to ASL: Identifying the influences of a self-generated childhood gesture system upon language proficiency in adulthood." In D. MacLaughlin & S. McEwen (Eds.), *Proceedings of the Nineteenth Boston University Conference on Language Development* (pp. 403–414). Somerville, MA: Cascadilla Press.

Morford, J. P., Singleton, J. L., & Goldin-Meadow, S. (1995b). "The genesis of language: How much time is needed to generate arbitrary symbols in a sign system?" In K. Emmorey & J. S. Reilly (Eds.), *Language, Gesture and Space* (pp. 313–332). Hillsdale, NJ: Lawrence Erlbaum Associates.

Morgan, B., Maybery, M., & Durkin, K. (2003). "Weak central coherence, poor joint attention and low verbal ability: Independent deficits in early autism." *Developmental Psychology, 39,* 646–656.

Mundy, P., Kasari, C., Sigman, M., & Ruskin, E. (1995). "Nonverbal communication and early language acquisition in children with Down syndrome and in normally developing children." *Journal of Speech and Hearing Research, 38,* 157–167.

Mundy, P., Sigman, M., & Kasari, C. (1990). "A longitudinal study of joint attention and language development in autistic children." *Journal of Autism and Developmental Disorders, 20,* 115–128.

Murphy, M. M. & Abbeduto, L. (2003). "Language and communication in fragile X syndrome." In L. Abbeduto (Ed.), *International Review of Research in Mental Retardation, Vol. 27* (pp. 83–119). New York: Academic Press.

Murphy, M. M. & Abbeduto, L. (2005). "Indirect genetic effects and the early language development of children with genetic mental retardation syndromes: The role of joint attention." *Infants and Young Children, 18,* 47–59.

Murphy, M. M., Abbeduto, L., Giles, N., Bruno, L., Richmond, E. K., & Schroeder, S. (2004). "Cognitive, language and social-cognitive skills of individuals with fragile X syndrome with and without autism." Poster presented at the annual Gatlinburg Conference on Mental Retardation, San Diego, CA.

Musselman, C. R., Wilson, A. K., & Lindsay, P. H. (1988). "Effects of early intervention on hearing impaired children." *Exceptional Children, 55*(3), 222–228.

Nass, R., Gross, A., & Devinsky, O. (1998). "Autism and autistic epileptiform regression with occipital spikes." *Developmental Medicine and Child Neurology, 40,* 453–458.

Nazzi, T. & Karmiloff-Smith, A. (2002). "Early categorization abilities in young children with Williams syndrome." *NeuroReport, 13*, 1259–1262.

Nazzi, T., Paterson, S., & Karmiloff-Smith, A. (2003). "Early word segmentation by infants and toddlers with Williams syndrome." *Infancy, 4*(2), 251–271.

Nespoulous, J. (1999). "Universal vs. language-specific constraints in agrammatic aphasia: Is comparatism back?" In C. Fuchs & S. Robert (Eds.), *Language Diversity and Cognitive Representations* (pp. 195–207). Amsterdam: John Benjamins.

Neville, H. J., Mills, D. L., & Bellugi, U. (1994). "Effects of altered auditory sensitivity and age of language acquisition on the development of language–relevant neural systems: Preliminary studies of Williams syndrome." In S. Broman & J. Grafman (Eds.), *Atypical Cognitive Deficits in Developmental Disorders: Implications for brain function* (pp. 67–83). Hillsdale, NJ: Lawrence Erlbaum Associates.

Newbury, D. & Monaco, A. (2002). "Molecular genetics of speech and language disorders." *Current Opinion in Pediatrics, 14*, 696–701.

Newport, E. L. (1990). "Maturational constraints on language learning." *Cognitive Science, 14*, 11–28.

Newport, E. L. (1991). "Contrasting conceptions of the critical period for language." In S. Carey & R. Gelman (Eds.), *The epigenesis of mind: Essays on biology and cognition* (pp. 111–130). Hillsdale, NJ: Lawrence Erlbaum Associates.

Newport, E. L., Bavelier, D., & Neville, H. J. (2001). "Critical thinking about critical periods: Perspectives on a critical period for language acquisition." In E. Dupoux (Ed.), *Language, Brain and Cognitive Development* (pp. 482–502). Cambridge, MA: The MIT Press.

Nicholas, J. G., & Geers, A. E. (2003). "Hearing status, language modality and young children's communicative and linguistic behavior." *Journal of Deaf Studies and Deaf Education, 8*, 422–437.

Nicholas, J. G. & Geers, A. E. (in press). "The process and early outcomes of cochlear implantation by three years of age." In P. E. Spencer & M. Marschark (Eds.), *Advances in the Spoken Language Development of Deaf Children.* New York: Oxford University Press.

Norbury, C. F., Bishop, D. V. M., & Briscoe, J. (2001). "Production of English finite verb morphology: A comparison of SLI and mild-moderate hearing impairment." *Journal of Speech, Language and Hearing Research, 44*, 165–178.

Nordin, V. & Gillberg, C. (1998). "The long-term course of autistic disorders: Update on follow-up studies." *Acta Psychiatrica Scandinavica, 97*, 99–108.

O'Hara, M. & Johnston, J. (1997). "Syntactic bootstrapping in children with specific language impairment." *European Journal of Disorders of Communication, 32*, 189–205.

O'Brien, E., Zhang, X., Nishimura, C., Tomblin, J., & Murray, J. (2003). "Association of specific language impairment (SLI) to the region of 7q31." *The American Journal of Human Genetics, 72*, 1536–1543.

O'Donoghue, G. M., Nikolopoulos, T. P., & Archbold, S. M. (2000). "Determinants of speech perception in children after cochlear implantation." *The Lancet, 356*, 762–767.

O'Donoghue, G. M., Nikolopoulos, T. P., Archbold, S. M., & Tait, M. (1999). "Cochlear implants in young children: The relationship between speech perception and speech intelligibility." *Ear and Hearing, 20*(5), 419–425.

Oller, D. K. (1980). "The emergence of the sounds of speech in infancy." In G. H. Yeni-Komshian, J. F. Kavanagh, & C. A. Ferguson (Eds.), *Child phonology, 1* (pp. 93–112). New York: Academic Press.

Oller, D. K. & Eilers, R. E. (1988). "The role of audition in infant babbling." *Child Development, 59*, 441–449.

Oostra, B. A. (1996). "FMR1 protein studies and animal models for fragile X syndrome." In R. J. Hagerman & A. C. Cronister (Eds.), *Fragile X Syndrome: Diagnosis, treatment and research* (2nd edition, pp. 193–209). Baltimore, MD: Johns Hopkins University Press.

Oostra, B. A. & Willemsen, R. (2003). "A fragile balance: FMR1 expression levels." *Human Molecular Genetics, 12*, Review Issue 2, R249–R257.

Osberger, M. J. & McGarr, N. S. (1982). "Speech production characteristics of the hearing impaired." In N. Lass (Ed.), *Speech and Language: Advances in basic research and practice* (pp. 257–316). New York: Academic Press.

Osberger, M. J., Maso, M., & Sam, L. K. (1993). "Speech intelligibility of children with cochlear implants, tactile aids, or hearing aids." *Journal of Speech and Hearing Research, 36*, 186–203.

Osberger, M. J., Miyamoto, R. T., Zimmerman-Phillips, S., Kemink, J. L., Stroer, B. S., Firszt, J. B., & Novak, M. A. (1991a). "Independent evaluation of the speech perception abilities of children with the Nucleus 22-channel cochlear implant system." *Ear and Hearing, 12*, 66–80.

Osberger, M. J., Robbins, A. M., Berry, S. W., Todd, S. L., Hesketh, L. J., & Sedey, A. (1991b). "Analysis of the spontaneous speech samples of children with cochlear implants or tactile aids." *The American Journal of Otology, 12*, 151–164.

Osberger, M. J., Robbins, A. M., Todd, S. L., & Riley, A. I. (1994). "Speech intelligibility of children with cochlear implants." *The Volta Review, 96*(5), 169–180.

Paterson, S. J. (2000). The Development of Language and Number Understanding in Williams Syndrome and Down's Syndrome: Evidence from the infant and mature phenotypes. Unpublished Ph.D. dissertation, University College London.

Paterson, S. J., Brown, J. H., Gsödl, M. K., Johnson, M. H., & Karmiloff-Smith, A. (1999). "Cognitive modularity and genetic disorders." *Science, 286*, 2355–2358.

Paul, R. & Cohen, D. (1984). "Responses to contingent queries in adults with mental retardation and pervasive developmental disorders." *Applied Psycholinguistics, 5*, 349–357.

Paul, R. & Cohen, D. (1985). "Comprehension of indirect requests in adults with mental retardation and pervasive developmental disorders." *Journal of Speech and Hearing Research, 28*, 475–479.

Paul, R., Cohen, D. J., Breg, R., Watson, M., & Herman, S. (1984). "Fragile X syndrome: Its relations to speech and language disorders." *Journal of Speech and Hearing Disorders, 49*, 326–336.

Paul, R., Dykens, E., Leckman, F., Watson, M., Breg, W. R., & Cohen, D. J. (1987). "A comparison of language characteristics of mentally retarded adults with fragile X syndrome and those with nonspecific mental retardation and autism." *Journal of Autism and Developmental Disorders, 17*, 457–468.

Paul, R., Fischer, M., & Cohen, D. (1988). "Brief report: Sentence comprehension strategies in children with autism and specific language disorders." *Journal of Autism and Developmental Disorders, 18*, 669–679.

Peters, A. (1997). "Typology, prosody and the acquisition of morphemes." In D. I. Slobin (Ed.), *The Cross-linguistic Study of Language Acquisition, Vol. 5* (pp. 135–197). Mahwah, NJ: Lawrence Erlbaum Associates.

Peña, E., Gutierrez-Clellen, V., Iglesias, A., Goldstein, B., & Bedore, L. M. (in preparation). "Bilingual English Spanish assessment (BESA)."

Pezzini, G, Vicari, S., Volterra, V., Milani, L., & Ossella, M. T. (1999). "Children with Williams syndrome: Is there a single neuropsychological profile?" *Developmental Neuropsychology, 15*, 141–155.

Phillips, C. E., Jarrold, C., Baddeley, A., Grant, J., & Karmiloff-Smith, A. (2004). "Comprehension of spatial language terms in Williams syndrome: Evidence for an interaction between domains of strength and weakness." *Cortex, 40*, 85–101.

Philofsky, A., Hepburn, S. L., Hayes, A., Hagerman, R., & Rogers, S. J. (2004). "Linguistic and cognitive functioning and autism symptoms in young children with fragile X syndrome." *American Journal on Mental Retardation, 109*, 208–218.

Piattelli-Palmarini, M. (2001). "Grammar – the basest essentials." *Nature, 411*, 887–888.

Pinker, S. (1989). *Learnability and Cognition: The acquisition of argument structure.* Cambridge, MA: The MIT Press.

Pinker, S. (1991). "Rules of language." *Science, 253*, 530–535.

Pinker, S. (1994). *The Language Instinct.* New York: W. Morrow and Co.

Pisoni, D. B., Cleary, M., Geers, A. E., & Tobey, E. A. (1999). "Individual differences in effectiveness of cochlear implants in children who are prelingually deaf: New process measures of performance." *The Volta Review, 101*(3), 111–164.

Plante, E. & Vance, R. (1994). "Selection of preschool language tests: A data-based approach." *Language, Speech, and Hearing Services in Schools, 25*, 15–24.

Prizant, B. (1983). "Language acquisition and communicative behavior in autism: toward an understanding of the "whole" of it." *Journal of Speech and Hearing Disorders, 48*, 296–307.

Prizant, B. & Rydell, P. (1993). "Assessment and intervention considerations for unconventional verbal behavior." In J. Reichle & D. Wacker (Eds.), *Communicative Alternatives to Challenging Behavior: Integrating functional assessment and intervention strategies* (pp. 263–297). Baltimore, MD: Brookes.

Prouty, L. A., Rogers, R. C., Stevenson, R. E., Dean, J. H., Palmer, K. K., Simensen, R. J., Coston, G. N., & Schwartz, C. E. (1988). "Fragile X syndrome: Growth, development and intellectual function." *American Journal of Medical Genetics, 30*, 123–142.

Pueschel, S. M. (1996). "Young people with Down syndrome: Transition from childhood to adulthood." *Mental Retardation and Developmental Disabilities Research Reviews, 2*, 90–95.

Quirk, R., Greenbaum, S., Leech, G., & Svartvik, J. (1972). *A Grammar of Contemporary English.* London: Longman.

Rapin, I. & Wilson, B. (1978). "Children with developmental language disability: Neurological aspects and assessment." In M. A. Wyke (Ed.), *Developmental Dysphasia* (pp. 13–41). London: Academic Press.

Reeves, R., Baxter, L., & Richtsmeier, J. (2001). "Too much of a good thing: Mechanisms of gene action in Down syndrome." *Trends in Genetics, 17*, 83–88.

Reilly, J., Losh, M., Bellugi, U., & Wulfeck, B. (2004). "'Frog, where are you?' Narratives in children with specific language impairment, early focal brain injury, and Williams syndrome." *Brain and Language, 88*, 229–242.

Reiss, A. L., Eckert, M. A., Rose, F. E., Karchemskiy, A., Kesler, S., Chang, M., Reynolds, M. F., Kwon, H., & Galaburda, A. (2004). "An experiment of nature: Brain anatomy parallels cognition and behaviour in Williams syndrome." *Journal of Neuroscience, 24*(21), 5009–5015.

Reynell, J. K. (1969). *Reynell Developmental Language Scales*. Slough, Bucks: NFER-Nelson Publishing.

Rice, M. (2004). "Growth models of developmental language disorders." In M. L. Rice & S. F. Warren (Eds.), *Developmental Language Disorders: From phenotypes to etiologies* (pp. 207–240). Mahwah, NJ: Lawrence Erlbaum Associates.

Rice, M., Buhr, J., & Nemeth, M. (1990). "Fast-mapping word-learning abilities of language-delayed preschoolers." *Journal of Speech and Hearing Disorders, 55*, 33–42.

Rice, M. & Wexler, K. (2001). *Rice/Wexler Test of Early Grammatical Impairment*. San Antonio, TX: Harcourt Assessment Inc.

Robbins, A. M., Bollard, P. M., & Green, J. (1999). "Language development in children implanted with the Clarion cochlear implant." *Annals of Otology, Rhinology and Laryngology, 108*, 113–118.

Robbins, A. M., Kirk, K. I., Osberger, M. J., & Ertmer, D. (1995). "Speech intelligibility of implanted children." *Annals of Otology, Rhinology and Laryngology, 166*, 399–401.

Robbins, A. M., Svirsky, M., & Kirk, K. I. (1997). "Children with implants can speak, but can they communicate?" *Archives of Otolaryngology, Head and Neck Surgery, 117*, 155–160.

Roberts, J. (1989). "Echolalia and comprehension in autistic children." *Journal of Autism and Developmental Disorders, 19*, 271–281.

Roberts, J. E., Mirrett, P., & Burchinal, M. (2001). "Receptive and expressive communication development of young males with fragile X syndrome." *American Journal on Mental Retardation, 106*, 216–230.

Robinshaw, H. M. (1996). "Acquisition of speech, pre- and post-cochlear implantation: Longitudinal studies of a congenitally deaf infant." *European Journal of Disorders of Communication, 31*, 121–139.

Robinson, K. (1998). "Implications of developmental plasticity for the language acquisition of deaf children with cochlear implants." *International Journal of Pediatric Otorhinolaryngology, 46*, 71–80.

Roizen, N. J. (2001). "Down syndrome: Progress in research." *Mental Retardation and Developmental Disabilities Research Reviews, 7*, 38–44.

Rosen, S. (2003). "Auditory processing in dyslexia and specific language impairment: Is there a deficit? What is its nature? Does it explain anything?" *Journal of Phonetics, 31*(3–4), 509–527.

Rosenberg, S. & Abbeduto, L. (1993). *Language and communication in mental retardation: Development, processes and intervention*. Hillsdale, NJ: Lawrence Erlbaum Associates.

Rosin, M. M., Swift, E., Bless, D., & Vetter, D. K. (1988). "Communication profiles of adolescents with Down syndrome." *Journal of Childhood Communication Disorders, 12*, 49–64.

Rossen, M., Klima, E. S., Bellugi, U., Bihrle, A., & Jones, W. (1996). "Interaction between language and cognition: Evidence from Williams syndrome." In J. H. Beitchman, N. Cohen, M. Konstantareas, & R. Tannock (Eds.), *Language Learning and Behaviour* (pp. 367–392). New York: Cambridge University Press.

Rossi, P. G., Parmeggiani, A., Posar, A., Scaduto, M. C., Chiodo, S., & Vatti, G. (1999). "Landau-Kleffner syndrome (LKS): Long-term follow-up and links with electrical status epilepticus during sleep (ESES)." *Brain and Development, 21*, 90–98.

Rowland, C. Pine, J., Lieven, E., & Theakston, A. (2003). "Determinants of acquisition order in wh-questions: Re-evaluating the role of caregiver speech." *Journal of Child Language, 30*, 609–635.

Ruben, R. (1997). "A time frame of critical/sensitive periods of language development." *Acta Otolaryngologica, 117*, 202–205.

Ruscio, J. & Ruscio, A. (2000). "Informing the continuity controversy: A taxometric analysis of depression." *Journal of Abnormal Psychology, 109*, 473–487.

Rutter, M., Greenfield, D., & Lockyer, L. (1967). "A five to fifteen year follow-up study of infantile psychosis: II. Social and behavioral outcome." *British Journal of Psychology and Psychiatry, 133*, 1183–1199.

Rydell, P. & Mirenda, P. (1994). "Effects of high and low constraint utterances on the production of immediate and delayed echolalia in young children with autism." *Journal of Autism and Developmental Disorders, 24*, 719–735.

Scarborough, H. S. (1990). "Index of productive syntax." *Applied Psycholinguistics, 11*, 1–22.

Schauwers, K., Gillis, S., Daemers, K., De Beukelaer, C., & Govaerts, P. J. (2004). "Cochlear implantation between 5 and 20 months of age: The onset of babbling and the audiological outcome." *Otology and Neurotology, 25*, 263–270.

Schiefelbusch, R. L. (1972). *Language of the Mentally Retarded.* Baltimore, MD: University Park Press.

Schiefelbusch, R. L. & Lloyd, L. L. (Eds.). (1974). *Language Perspectives – Acquisition, Retardation, and Intervention.* Baltimore, MD: University Park Press.

Sehgal, S. T., Kirk, K. I., Svirsky, M., Ertmer, D. J., & Osberger, M. J. (1998). "Imitative consonant feature production by children with multichannel sensory aids." *Ear and Hearing, 19*, 72–84.

Seibert, J. M., Hogan, A. E., & Mundy, P. C. (1982). "Assessing interactional competencies: The early social-communication scales." *Infant Mental Health Journal, 3*, 244–258.

Seidenberg, M. S. (2003). "Critical periods in language and other domains: The paradox of success." Paper presented at the Society for Research in Child Development, Tampa, FL.

Semel, E. & Rosner, S. R. (2003). *Understanding Williams syndrome: Behavioral patterns and interventions.* Mahwah, NJ: Lawrence Erlbaum Associates.

Semel, E., Wiig, E., & Secord, W. (1987). *Clinical Evaluation of Language Fundamentals* (3rd edition). San Antonio, TX: The Psychological Corporation, Harcourt Brace and Co.

Serry, T. A. & Blamey, P. J. (1999). "A 4-year investigation into phonetic inventory development in young cochlear implant users." *Journal of Speech, Language and Hearing Research, 42*, 141–154.

Serry, T. A., Blamey, P., & Grogan, M. (1997). "Phoneme acquisition in the first 4 years of implant use." *The American Journal of Otology, 18*, 122–124.

Seung, H.-K. & Chapman, R. S. (2000). "Digit span in individuals with Down syndrome and typically developing children: Temporal aspects." *Journal of Speech, Language and Hearing Research, 43*, 609–620.

Seymour, H., Roeper, T., & de Villiers, J. (2003). *Diagnostic Evaluation of Language Variation: Screening Test.* San Antonio, TX: The Psychological Corporation.

Sharma, A., Dorman, M., & Spohr, A. (2002a). "Early cochlear implantation in children allows normal development of central auditory pathways." *Annals of Otology, Rhinology and Laryngology, 111*, 38–41.

Sharma, A., Dorman, M., & Spohr, A. (2002b). "Rapid development of cortical auditory evoked potentials after early cochlear implantation." *NeuroReport, 13*, 1346–1368.

Shinnar, S., Rapin, I., Arnold, S., Tuchman, R., Shulman, L., Ballaban-Gil, K., Maw, M., Deuel, R. K., & Volkmar, F. R. (2001). "Language regression in childhood." *Pediatric Neurology, 24*, 183–189.

Silverman, W. & Wisniewski, H. M. (1999). "Down syndrome and Alzheimer disease: Variability in individual vulnerability." In J. A. Rondal & L. Nadel (Eds.), *Down Syndrome: A review of current knowledge* (pp. 178–194). London: Whurr Publishers.

Singer Harris, N. G., Bellugi, U., Bates, E., Jones, W., & Rossen, M. (1997). "Contrasting profiles of language development in children with Williams and Down syndromes." *Developmental Neuropsychology, 13*, 345–370.

Siple, P., Caccamise, F., & Brewer, L. (1982). "Signs as pictures and signs as words: Effect of language knowledge on memory for new vocabulary." *Journal of Experimental Psychology: Language, memory and cognition, 8*, 619–625.

Skinner, B. F. (1957). *Verbal Behavior.* New York: Appleton-Century-Crofts.

Smith, C. R. (1975). "Residual hearing and speech production in deaf children." *Journal of Speech and Hearing Research, 18*, 795–811.

Smith, N. & Tsimpli, I. (1995). *The Mind of a Savant: Language learning and modularity.* Oxford: Blackwell.

Snik, A. F. M., Vermeulen, A. M., Geelen, C. P. L., Brokx, J. P. L., & van der Broek, P. (1997). "Speech perception performance of congenitally deaf patients with a cochlear implant: The effect of age at implantation." *The American Journal of Otology, 18*, 138–139.

Spencer, L. J., Tye-Murray, N., & Tomblin, J. B. (1998). "The production of English inflectional morphology, speech production and listening performance in children with cochlear implants." *Ear and Hearing, 19*, 310–318.

Spencer, P. E. (1993). "The expressive communication of hearing mothers and deaf infants." *American Annals of the Deaf, 138*(3), 275–283.

Spencer, P. E. (in press). "Individual differences in language performance after cochlear implantation at one to three years of age: Child, family and linguistic factors." *Journal of Deaf Studies and Deaf Education.*

Spencer, P. E. & Lederberg, A. R. (1997). "Different modes, different models: Communication and language of young deaf children and their mothers." In L. B. Adamson & M. A. Romski (Eds.), *Research on Communication and Language Disorders: Contributions to theories of language development* (pp. 203–230). Baltimore, MD: Brookes Publishing Co.

Spencer, P. E. & Marschark, M. (2003). "Cochlear implants: Issues and implications." In M. Marschark & P. E. Spencer (Eds.), *Oxford Handbook of Deaf Studies, Language and Education* (pp. 434–449). New York: Oxford University Press.

Stark, R. & Montgomery, J. (1995). "Sentence processing in language-impaired children under conditions of filtering and time compression." *Applied Psycholinguistics, 16*, 137–154.

Stark, R. E. (1980). "Stages of speech development in the first year of life." In G. H. Yeni-Komshian, J. F. Kavanagh, & C. A. Ferguson (Eds.), *Child Phonology, 1* (pp. 73–92). New York: Academic Press.

Stark, R. E. (1983). "Phonatory development in young normally hearing and hearing-impaired children." In H. Hochberg, H. Levitt, & M. J. Osberger (Eds.), *Speech of the Hearing-impaired: Research, training and personnel preparation* (pp. 297–312). Baltimore, MD: University Park.

Steele, S., Joseph, R., & Tager-Flusberg, H. (2003). "Brief report: Developmental change in theory of mind abilities in children with autism." *Journal of Autism and Developmental Disorders, 33*, 461–467.

Stevens, T. & Karmiloff-Smith, A. (1997). "Word learning in a special population: Do individuals with Williams syndrome obey lexical constraints?" *Journal of Child Language, 24*, 737–765.

Stoel-Gammon, C. (1988). "Prelinguistic vocalizations of hearing-impaired and normally hearing subjects: A comparison of consonantal inventories." *Journal of Speech and Hearing Disorders, 53*, 302–315.

Stoel-Gammon, C. (1997). "Phonological development in Down syndrome." *Mental Retardation and Developmental Disabilities Research Review, 3*, 300–306.

Stoel-Gammon, C. & Otomo, K. (1986). "Babbling development of hearing-impaired and normally hearing subjects." *Journal of Speech and Hearing Disorders, 51*, 33–41.

Stojanovik, V., Perkins, M., & Howard, S. (2004). "Williams syndrome and specific language impairment do not support developmental double dissociations and innate modularity." *Journal of Neurolinguistics, 17*, 403–489.

Stokes, S. F. (2002). "Lexical and morphological diversity in children with SLI: Evidence in support of an optionality constraint." Paper presented at IASCL-SRCLD, July, Madison, WI.

Stokes, S. F. & Fletcher, P. (2000). "Lexical diversity and productivity in Cantonese-speaking children with specific language impairment." *International Journal of Language and Communication Disorders, 35*, 527–541.

Stokes, S. F. & Fletcher, P. (2003). "Aspect markers in Cantonese-speaking children with specific language impairment." *Linguistics, 41*, 381–406.

Stokes, S. F., Fletcher, P., & Leung, S. (1997). *Language Development in Cantonese-speaking Children with Specific Language Impairment.* Hong Kong: Hong Kong Research Grants Council.

Stone, W. L. & Yoder, P. J. (2001). "Predicting spoken language level in children with autism spectrum disorders." *Autism, 5*, 341–346.

Stores, R., Stores, G., Fellows, B., & Buckley, S. (1998). "Daytime behaviour problems and maternal stress in children with Down's syndrome, their siblings and non-intellectually disabled and other intellectually disabled peers." *Journal of Intellectual Disabilities Research, 42*, 228–237.

Sudhalter, V., Cohen, I. L., Silverman, W., & Wolf-Schein, E. G. (1990). "Conversational analyses of males with fragile X, Down syndrome and autism: Comparison of the emergence of deviant language." *American Journal on Mental Retardation, 94*, 431–441.

Sudhalter, V., Scarborough, H. S., & Cohen, I. L. (1991). "Syntactic delay and pragmatic deviance in the language of fragile X males." *American Journal of Medical Genetics, 38*, 493–497.

Svirsky, M. A., Teoh, S., & Neuburger, H. (in press). "Development of language and speech perception in congenitally, profoundly deaf children as a function of age at cochlear implantation." *Audiology and Neuro-Otology.*

Svirsky, M. A., Chute, P. M., Green, J., Bollard, P., & Miyamoto, R. T. (2000). "Language development in children who are prelingually deaf who have used the SPEAK or CIS stimulation strategies since initial stimulation." *The Volta Review, 102*(4), 199–213.

Svirsky, M. A., Robbins, A. M., Kirk, K. I., Pisoni, D. B., & Miyamoto, R. T. (2000). "Language development in profoundly deaf children with cochlear implants." *Psychological Science, 11*(2), 153–158.

Svirsky, M. A., Stallings, L. M., Lento, C. L., Ying, E., & Leonard, L. B. (2002). "Grammatical morphologic development in pediatric cochlear implant users may be affected by the perceptual prominence of the relevant markers." *Annals of Otology, Rhinology and Laryngology, 111*(5), 109–112.

Swisher, M. V. & Christie, K. (1989). "Communication using a signed code for English: Interaction between deaf children and their mothers." *Monographs for the International Sign Linguistics Association Centre for Deaf Studies, 1*, 36–44.

Szagun, G. (1997). "Some aspects of language development in normal-hearing children and children with cochlear implants." *The American Journal of Otology, 18*, 131–134.

Szagun, G. (2000). "The acquisition of grammatical and lexical structures in children with cochlear implants: A developmental psycholinguistic approach." *Audiology and Neuro-Otology, 5*, 39–47.

Szagun, G. (2001). "Language acquisition in young German-speaking children using cochlear implants: Individual differences and implications of a 'sensitive phase'." *Audiology and Neuro-Otology, 6*(5), 288–297.

Tager-Flusberg, H. (1997). "The role of theory of mind in language acquisition: Contributions from the study of autism." In L. Adamson & M. A. Romski (Eds.), *Communication and Language Acquisition: Discoveries from atypical development* (pp. 133–158). Baltimore, MD: Brookes.

Tager-Flusberg, H. (1999). "A psychological approach to understanding the social and language impairments in autism." *International Review of Psychiatry, 11*, 325–334.

Tager-Flusberg, H. (2000). "Language and understanding minds: Connections in autism." In S. Baron-Cohen, H. Tager-Flusberg, & D. J. Cohen (Eds.), *Understanding Other Minds: Perspectives from developmental cognitive neuroscience* (2nd edition, pp. 124–149). Oxford: Oxford University Press.

Tager-Flusberg, H. & Cooper, J. (1999). "Present and future possibilities for defining a phenotype for specific language impairment." *Journal of Speech, Language, and Hearing Research, 42*, 1275–1278.

Tager-Flusberg, H. & Joseph, R. M. (in press). "How language facillitates the acquisition of false belief in children with autism." In J. Astington & J. Baird (Eds.), *Why Language Matters for Theory of Mind*. Oxford: Oxford University Press.

Tager-Flusberg, H. & Sullivan, K. (1994). "Predicting and explaining behavior: A comparison of autistic, mentally retarded and normal children." *Journal of Child Psychology and Psychiatry, 35*, 1059–1075.

Tager-Flusberg, H. & Sullivan, K. (1997). "Early language development in children with mental retardation." In E. J. Burack, R. Hodapp, & E. Zigler (Eds.), *Handbook of Development and Retardation* (pp. 208–239). New York: Cambridge University Press.

Tager-Flusberg, H., Plesa-Skwerer, D., Faja, S., & Joseph, R. M. (2003). "People with Williams syndrome process faces holistically." *Cognition, 89*, 11–24.

Tager-Flusberg, H., Calkins, S., Nolin, T., Baumberger, T., Anderson, M., & Chadwick-Dias, A. (1990). "A longitudinal study of language acquisition in autistic and Down syndrome children." *Journal of Autism and Developmental Disorders, 20*, 1–21.

Tait, D. M. (1993). "Video analysis: A method of assessing changes in preverbal and early linguistic communication after cochlear implantation." *Ear and Hearing, 14*(6), 378–389.

Tait, D. M. & Lutman, M. E. (1994). "Comparison of early communicative behavior in young children with cochlear implants and with hearing aids". *Ear and Hearing, 15*, 352–361.

Tait, D. M., Lutman, M. E., & Robinson, K. (2000). "Preimplant measures of preverbal communicative behavior as predictors of cochlear implant outcomes in children." *Ear and Hearing, 21*, 18–24.

Tallal, P. & Piercy, M. (1978). "Defects of auditory perception in children with developmental dysphasia." In M. A. Wyke (Ed.), *Developmental Dysphasia* (pp. 63–84). London: Academic Press.

Temple, C., Almazan, M., & Sherwood, S. (2002). "Lexical skills in Williams syndrome: A cognitive neuropsychological analysis." *Journal of Neurolinguistics, 15*(6), 463–495.

Thomas, M. S. C. (2003). "Limits on plasticity." *Journal of Cognition and Development, 4*(1), 95–121.

Thomas, M. S. C. (2005). "Characterising compensation." *Cortex, 41*, 434–440.

Thomas, M. S. C. (in press). "Williams syndrome: Fractionations all the way down?: Commentary on Semel and Rosner." *Cortex*.

Thomas, M. S. C. & Karmiloff-Smith, A. (2002a). "Are developmental disorders like cases of adult brain damage? Implications from connectionist modelling." *Behavioural and Brain Sciences, 25*(6), 727–780.

Thomas, M. S. C. & Karmiloff-Smith, A. (2002b). "Modelling typical and atypical cognitive development." In U. Goswami (Ed.), *Handbook of Childhood Development* (pp. 575–599). Oxford: Blackwell.

Thomas, M. S. C. & Karmiloff-Smith, A. (2003). "Modelling language acquisition in atypical phenotypes." *Psychological Review, 110*(4), 647–682.

Thomas, M. S. C. & Redington, M. (2004). "Modelling atypical syntax processing." In W. Sakas (Ed.), *Proceedings of the COLING-2004 Workshop: Psycho-computational model of human language acquisition* (pp. 85–92). Geneva, Switzerland, August 2004.

Thomas, M. S. C. & Karmiloff-Smith, A. (2005). "Can developmental disorders reveal the component parts of the human language faculty?" *Language Learning and Development, 1*, 65–92.

Thomas, M. S. C. & Richardson, F. (in press). "Atypical representational change." To appear in *Proceeding of Attention and Performance XXI: Processes of change in brain and cognitive development.* Denver, CO.

Thomas, M. S. C., Dockrell, J. E., Messer, D., Parmigiani, C., Ansari, D., & Karmiloff-Smith, A. (submitted). "Naming in Williams syndrome."

Thomas, M. S. C., Grant, J., Gsödl, M., Laing, E., Barham, Z., Lakusta, L., Tyler, L. K., Grice, S., Paterson, S., & Karmiloff-Smith, A. (2001). "Past tense formation in Williams syndrome." *Language and Cognitive Processes, 16*, 143–176.

Thordardottir, E., Chapman, R. S., & Wagner, L. (2002). "Complex sentence use in children with Down Syndrome." *Applied Psycholinguistics, 24*, 163–183.

Thordardottir, E., Ellis Weismer, S., & Evans, J. (2002). "Continuity in lexical and morphological development in Icelandic and English-speaking 2-year olds." *First Language, 22*, 3–28.

Tingley, E. C., Gleason, J. B., & Hooshyar, N. (1994). "Mothers' lexicon of internal state words in speech to children with Down syndrome and to nonhandicapped children at mealtime." *Journal of Communication Disorders, 27*, 135–155.

Tjus, T., Heimann, M., & Nelson, K. E. (1998). "Gains in literacy through the use of a specially developed multimedia computer strategy: Positive findings from 13 children with autism." *Autism, 2*, 139–156.

Tobey, E. A. & Geers, A. E. (1995). "Speech production benefits of cochlear implants." *Advances in Otorhinolaryngology, 50*, 146–153.

Tobey, E. A., Geers, A. E., & Brenner, C. (1994). "Speech production results: Speech feature acquisition." *The Volta Review, 96*(5), 109–129.

Tobey, E. A. & Hasenstab, M. S. (1991). "Effects of a Nucleus multichannel cochlear implant upon speech production in children." *Ear and Hearing, 12*(4), 48–54.

Tobey, E. A., Angelette, S., Murchison, C., Nicosia, J., Sprague, S., Staller, S. J., Brimacombe, J. A., & Beiter, A. L. (1991). "Speech production performance in children with multichannel cochlear implants." *The American Journal of Otology, 12*, 165–173.

Tobey, E. A., Geers, A. E., Douek, B. M., Perrin, J., Skellett, R., Brenner, C., & Toretta, G. (2000). "Factors associated with speech intelligibility in children with cochlear implants." *Annals of Otology, Rhinology and Laryngology, 185*, 28–30.

Tobey, E. A., Pancamo, S., Staller, S. J., Brimacombe, J. A., & Beiter, A. L. (1991). "Consonant production in children receiving a multichannel cochlear implant." *Ear and Hearing, 12*(1), 23–31.

Tomasello, M. (1998). "The return of constructions." *Journal of Child Language, 25*, 431–442.

Tomasello, M. (2000a). "Acquiring syntax is not what you think." In D. V. M. Bishop & L. B. Leonard (Eds.), *Speech and Language Impairments in Children* (pp. 1–15). Hove: Psychology Press.

Tomasello, M. (2000b). "Do young children have adult syntactic competence?" *Cognition, 74*, 209–253.

Tomasello, M. (2003). *Constructing a Language: A usage-based theory of language acquisition.* Cambridge, MA: Harvard University Press.

Tomasello, M. & Brooks, P. (1998). "Young children's earliest transitive and intransitive constructions." *Cognitive Linguistics, 9*, 379–395.

Tomasello, M. & Stahl, A. (2004). "Sampling children's speech: How much is enough?" *Journal of Child Language, 31*, 101–121.

Tomblin, J., Hafeman, L., & O'Brien, M. (2003). "Autism and autism risk in siblings of children with specific language impairment." *International Journal of Language and Communication Disorders, 38*, 235–250.

Tomblin, J. B., Spencer, L., Flock, S., Tyler, R., & Gantz, B. (1999). "A comparison of language achievement in children with cochlear implants and children using hearing aids." *Journal of Speech, Language and Hearing Research, 42*, 497–511.

Tomblin, J. B., Records, N., Buckwalter, P., Zhang, X., Smith, E., & O'Brien, M. (1997). "Prevalence of specific language impairment in kindergarten children." *Journal of Speech, Language, and Hearing Research, 40*, 1245–1260.

Trask, R. L. (1993). *A Dictionary of Grammatical Terms in Linguistics.* London: Routledge.

Tuchman, R. F. (1997). "Acquired epileptiform aphasia." *Seminars in Pediatric Neurology, 4*, 93–102.

Tye-Murray, N. & Kirk, K. I. (1993). "Vowel and diphthong production by young users of cochlear implants and the relationship between the phonetic level evaluation and spontaneous speech." *Journal of Speech and Hearing Research, 36*, 488–502.

Tye-Murray, N., Spencer, L., & Woodworth, G. G. (1995). "Acquisition of speech by children who have prolonged cochlear implant experience." *Journal of Speech and Hearing Research, 38*, 327–337.

Tye-Murray, N., Spencer, L., Bedia, E. G., & Woodworth, G. (1996). "Differences in children's sound production when speaking with a cochlear implant turned on and turned off." *Journal of Speech and Hearing Research, 39*, 604–610.

Tyler, R. S., Fryauf-Bertschy, H., Kelsay, D. M. R., Gantz, B. J., Woodworth, G. P., & Parkinson, A. (1997). "Speech perception by prelingually deaf children using cochlear implants." *Archives of Otolaryngology, Head and Neck Surgery, 117*, 180–187.

Ullman, M. T. & Pierpont, E. I. (2005). "Specific language impairment is not specific to language: The Procedural Deficit Hypothesis." *Cortex, 41*, 399–433.

van der Lely, H. K. J. & Ullman, M. (1996). "The computation and representation of past tense morphology in normally developing and specifically language impaired children." *Proceedings of the Annual Boston University Conference on Language Development, 20*(2), 804–815.

van der Lely, H. K. J. & Ullman, M. T. (2001). "Past tense morphology in specially language impaired and normally developing children." *Language and Cognitive Processes, 16*, 177–217.

Vicari, S., Carlesimo, G., Brizzolara, D., & Pezzini, G. (1996). "Short-term memory in children with Williams syndrome: A reduced contribution of lexical-semantic knowledge to word span." *Neuropsychologia, 34*, 919–925.

Vicari, S., Caselli, M. C., & Tonucci, F. (2000). "Asynchrony of lexical and morphosyntactic development in children with Down syndrome." *Neuropsychologia, 38*, 634–644.

Vihman, M. M., Ferguson, C. A., & Elbert, M. (1986). "Phonological development from babbling to speech: Common tendencies and individual differences." *Applied Psycholinguistics, 7*, 3–40.

Volterra, V., Capirci, O., & Caselli, M. C. (2001). "What atypical populations can reveal about language development: The contrast between deafness and Williams syndrome." *Language and Cognitive Processes, 16*, 219–239.

Volterra, V., Capirci, O., Pezzini, G., Sabbadini, L., & Vicari, S. (1996). "Linguistic abilities in Italian children with Williams syndrome." *Cortex, 32*, 663–677.

Wagner, K. R. (1985). "How much do children say in a day?" *Journal of Child Language, 12*, 457–487.

Waller, N., Putnam, F., & Carlson, E. (1996). "Types of dissociation and dissociative types: A taxometric analysis of dissociative experiences." *Psychological Methods, 1*, 300–321.

Waltzman, S. B. & Cohen, N. L. (1998). "Cochlear implantation in children younger than 2 years old." *The American Journal of Otology, 19*, 158–162.

Waltzman, S. B., Cohen, N. L., Gomolin, R. H., Shapiro, W. H., Ozdamar, S. R., & Hoffman, R. A. (1994). "Long-term results of early cochlear implantation in congenitally and prelingually deafened children." *The American Journal of Otology, 15*, 9–13.

Waltzman, S. B., Cohen, N. L., Gomolin, R. H., Green, J. E., Shapiro, W. H., Hoffman, R. A., & Roland, J. T. (1997). "Open-set speech perception in congenitally deaf children using cochlear implants." *The American Journal of Otology, 18*, 342–349.

Warburton, P., Baird, G., Chen, W., Morris, K., Jacobs, B., Hodgson, S., & Docherty, Z. (2000). "Support for linkage of autism and specific language impairment to 7q3 from two chromosome rearrangements involving band 7q31." *American Journal of Medical Genetics, 96*, 228–234.

Webelhuth, G. (1995). "X-bar theory and case theory." In G. Webelhuth (Ed.), *Government and Binding Theory and the Minimalist Program* (pp. 18–95). Oxford: Blackwell.

Whitehurst, G. & Fischel, J. (2000). "Reading and language impairments in conditions of poverty." In D. Bishop & L. Leonard (Eds.), *Speech and Language Impairments in Children* (pp. 53–71). Hove: Psychology Press.

Wilkinson, K. & Mazzitelli, K. (2003). "The effect of 'missing' information on children's retention of fast-mapped labels." *Journal of Child, Language 30*, 47–73.

Williams, K. T. (1997). *Expressive Vocabulary Test.* Circle Pines, MN: American Guidance Service.

Wing, L. (1971). "Perceptual and language development in autistic children: A comparative study." In M. Rutter (Ed.), *Infantile Autism: Concepts, characteristics and treatment* (pp. 173–195). London: Churchill.

Wisbeck, J. M., Huffman, L. C., Freund, L., Gunnar, M., Davis, E. P., & Reiss, A. L. (2000). "Cortisol and social stressors in children with fragile X: A pilot study." *Developmental and Behavioral Pediatrics, 21*, 279–282.

Wishart, J. G. & Pitcairn, T. K. (2000). "Recognition of identity and expression in faces by children with Down syndrome." *American Journal on Mental Retardation, 105*, 466–479.

Wolf-Schein, E. G., Cohen, I. L., Fisch, G. S., Brown, W. T., & Jenkins, E. C. (1987). "Speech-language and the fragile X syndrome: Initial findings and directions for study." *Journal of the American Speech and Hearing Association, 29*, 35–38.

Wolk, L. & Edwards, M. L. (1993). "The emerging phonological system of an autistic child." *Journal of Communication Disorders, 26*, 161–177.

Wolk, L. & Giesen, J. (2000). "A phonological investigation of four siblings with childhood autism." *Journal of Communication Disorders, 33*, 371–389.

Wong, A. M.-Y., Leonard, L. Fletcher, P., & Stokes, S. (2004). "Questions without movement: a study of Cantonese-speaking children with and without language impairment." *Journal of Speech, Language and Hearing Research, 47*, 1440–1453.

Wong, A. M.-Y., Stokes, S. F., & Fletcher, P. (2003). "Collocational diversity in perfective aspect zo2 use in Cantonese children with SLI." *Journal of Multilingual Communication Disorders, 1*, 132–140.

World Health Organization. (1993). *Mental disorders: A glossary and guide to their classification in accordance with the 10th revision of the International Classification of Diseases: Research Diagnostic Criteria* (*ICD-10*). Geneva: Author.

Wright, M., Purcell, A., & Reed, V. A. (2002). "Cochlear implants and infants: Expectations and outcomes." *Annals of Otology, Rhinology and Laryngology, 111*, 131–137.

Yirmiya, N., Erel, O., Shaked, M., & Solomonica-Levi, D. (1998). "Meta-analyses comparing theory of mind abilities of individuals with autism, individuals with mental retardation and normally developing individuals." *Psychological Bulletin, 124*, 283–307.

Yoshinaga-Itano, C. & Snyder, L. S. (1985). "Form and meaning in the written language of hearing-impaired children." *The Volta Review, 87*, 775–790.

Yoshinaga-Itano, C., Sedey, A. L., Coulter, D. K., & Mehl, A. L. (1998). "Language of early- and late-identified children with hearing loss." *American Academy of Pediatrics, 102*(5), 1161–1171.

Zelazo, P. D., Burack, J. A., Benedetto, E., & Frye, D. (1996). "Theory of mind and rule use in individuals with Down's syndrome: a test of the uniqueness and specificity claims." *Journal of Child Psychology and Psychiatry, 37*, 479–484.

Zhang, X. & Tomblin, J. B. (in preparation). "Developmental language disorder: A categorical or dimensional construct?"

Zukowski, A. (2001). Uncovering Grammatical Competence in Children with Williams Syndrome. Unpublished Ph.D. dissertation, Boston University.

Author index

Subject index

In the series *Trends in Language Acquisition Research* the following titles have been published thus far or are scheduled for publication:

1 **CENOZ, Jasone and Fred GENESEE (eds.):** Trends in Bilingual Acquisition. 2001. viii, 288 pp.

2 **MORGAN, Gary and Bencie WOLL (eds.):** Directions in Sign Language Acquisition. 2002. xx, 339 pp.

3 **BERMAN, Ruth A. (ed.):** Language Development across Childhood and Adolescence. 2004. xiv, 308 pp.

4 **FLETCHER, Paul and Jon F. MILLER (eds.):** Developmental Theory and Language Disorders. 2005. x, 216 pp.